The Dr. Barbara Natural Healing Cookbook

Unlock Your Body's Healing Power with Wholesome Plant-Based Recipes Inspired by Barbara O'Neill's Teachings and a 28-Day Meal Plan

Daisy Bloom

BONUSES

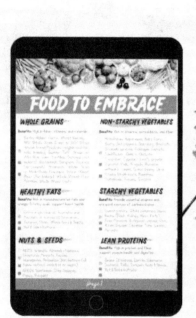

Healing Food Shopping Guide

Wellness Food Journal

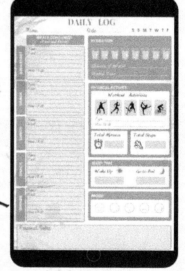

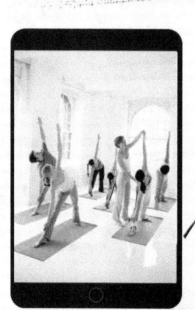

Natural Healing Yoga Flows Videos

...and a curated collection of Barbara O'Neill's insightful videos

Scroll to page 27, and SCAN the QR CODE!

Disclaimer

Table of Content

Introduction

Welcome to **"The Dr. Barbara's Natural Healing Cookbook"**. This book is your gateway to vibrant health and wellness through the power of wholesome, plant-based nutrition. Whether you're seeking to improve your energy levels, manage chronic conditions, or simply embrace a healthier lifestyle, you've come to the right place.

In this cookbook, you'll find a collection of delicious, easy-to-follow recipes inspired by the teachings of Barbara O'Neill, a renowned expert in natural healing and holistic health. Each recipe is designed to nourish your body, support your well-being, and help you unlock your body's natural healing power.

You'll also discover a comprehensive 28-day meal plan, practical tips for maintaining a healthy diet, and insightful information on the importance of whole foods, hydration, and natural remedies. Our goal is to provide you with the tools and knowledge you need to make lasting, positive changes to your health.

By choosing to explore the pages of this cookbook, you're taking a significant step toward a healthier, happier you. We hope this journey will inspire you to embrace the power of natural healing and enjoy the delicious benefits of plant-based eating.

About Barbara O'Neill

Barbara O'Neill is a leading figure in the field of natural healing and holistic health. With over three decades of experience, Barbara has dedicated her life to educating others about the transformative power of natural remedies and plant-based nutrition. She believes that the body has an innate ability to heal itself when given the right conditions, and her teachings emphasize the importance of a balanced diet, detoxification, and a holistic approach to health.

Barbara's journey into natural healing began with her own health challenges. Through extensive research and practical application, she discovered the profound impact that diet and lifestyle changes could have on her well-being. This personal experience ignited her passion for helping others achieve optimal health through natural means.

As a sought-after speaker and author, Barbara has shared her knowledge with countless individuals around the world. Her philosophy is grounded in the belief that true health is achieved by addressing the root causes of illness, rather than merely treating symptoms. She advocates for a diet rich in whole, unprocessed foods, regular detoxification, and the use of natural remedies to support the body's healing processes.

In this cookbook, we have compiled recipes and health tips that reflect Barbara O'Neill's holistic approach. Each recipe is crafted to provide maximum nutritional benefit, using ingredients that support the body's natural healing abilities. We hope that by incorporating these recipes into your daily routine, you will experience the profound benefits of a holistic, plant-based diet and take significant strides toward better health. Let's embark on this journey together, embracing the wisdom of Barbara O'Neill and the transformative power of wholesome, natural foods. Here's to your health and wellness!

Section I: Core Principles of Healing Nutrition

1. The Foundations of Holistic Health

1.1 Holistic Health Overview

Holistic health is a comprehensive approach to well-being that emphasizes the interconnectedness of the mind, body, and spirit. Unlike conventional medicine, which often focuses on treating symptoms, holistic health aims to address the root causes of illness and promote overall balance. This approach recognizes that health is more than just the absence of disease; it is a state of complete physical, mental, and social well-being.

One of the key principles of holistic health is the belief in the body's innate ability to heal itself. When given the right conditions—such as proper nutrition, adequate hydration, and a balanced lifestyle—the body can repair, regenerate, and thrive. This perspective challenges the conventional healthcare model and encourages individuals to take an active role in their health journey.

The benefits of holistic health are manifold. By treating the whole person rather than just the symptoms, holistic health practices can lead to improved energy levels, better mental clarity, enhanced emotional stability, and a greater sense of overall well-being. Additionally, holistic health approaches can help prevent chronic diseases, manage existing health conditions, and promote longevity.

1.2 Nutrition and Lifestyle

Role of Nutrition: Nutrition is a cornerstone of holistic health. The food we consume has a profound impact on our body's ability to function and heal. A diet rich in whole, unprocessed foods provides the essential nutrients our bodies need to thrive. These foods—fruits, vegetables, whole grains, nuts, seeds, and legumes—are packed with vitamins, minerals, antioxidants, and phytochemicals that support overall health and prevent disease.

In holistic nutrition, the focus is on eating a balanced, plant-based diet that minimizes processed foods and artificial additives. This approach not only nourishes the body but also helps in detoxification, supports the immune system, and enhances mental clarity. Barbara O'Neill advocates for mindful eating, emphasizing the importance of choosing foods that are close to their natural state and free from harmful chemicals.

Lifestyle Factors: Lifestyle choices play a crucial role in holistic health. Regular physical activity, sufficient sleep, stress management, and meaningful social connections are all vital components of a healthy lifestyle. Engaging in activities like yoga, meditation, and outdoor exercise can help reduce stress, improve mood, and boost physical health.

Natural Remedies: Holistic health often incorporates natural remedies and alternative therapies to support the body's healing processes. These can include herbal medicine, acupuncture, aromatherapy, and massage therapy. Such practices are used not only to treat specific health issues but also to maintain overall balance and prevent illness.

Detoxification: Detoxification is another essential aspect of holistic health. The body accumulates toxins from various sources, including the environment, food, and stress. Regular detox practices—such as fasting, juicing, and consuming detoxifying foods—can help eliminate these toxins and rejuvenate the body's systems. Barbara O'Neill emphasizes the importance of periodic detoxification to maintain optimal health and vitality.

Hydration: Proper hydration is fundamental to holistic health. Water is essential for nearly every bodily function, from digestion and nutrient absorption to temperature regulation and detoxification. Drinking clean, filtered water throughout the day ensures that the body's cells remain hydrated and function optimally. Barbara O'Neill recommends starting the day with a glass of warm lemon water to kickstart digestion and support detoxification.

2. Understanding Whole Foods and Plant-Based Nutrition

Whole, unprocessed foods are the cornerstone of a healthy diet and a key component of holistic health. These foods, which have been minimally altered from their natural state, provide a wealth of essential nutrients that support the body's natural functions. By consuming whole foods, you can enjoy a range of health benefits that contribute to overall well-being.

2.1 Benefits of Consuming Whole Foods

Nutrient Density: Whole foods are rich in essential vitamins, minerals, antioxidants, and fiber. Unlike processed foods, which often lose nutrients during manufacturing, whole foods retain their nutritional integrity. For example, fruits and vegetables are packed with antioxidants that help combat oxidative stress and reduce inflammation. Whole grains provide sustained energy and support digestive health, while nuts and seeds offer healthy fats crucial for brain function and hormone balance.

Improved Digestion: The fiber in whole foods promotes healthy digestion by aiding in the smooth passage of food through the digestive tract. This can help prevent constipation, reduce the risk of developing diverticulitis, and support a healthy gut microbiome. A diet rich in fiber can also help regulate blood sugar levels and promote a feeling of fullness, aiding in weight management.

Enhanced Immune Function: Whole foods contain a variety of nutrients that strengthen the immune system. Vitamins such as C, D, and E, along with minerals like zinc and selenium, play crucial roles in maintaining immune health. By incorporating a diverse range of whole foods into your diet, you can provide your body with the tools it needs to fend off infections and diseases.

Reduced Risk of Chronic Diseases: Consuming a diet rich in whole foods has been linked to a lower risk of developing chronic diseases such as heart disease, diabetes, and certain cancers. The antioxidants, phytochemicals, and anti-inflammatory compounds found in whole foods help protect cells from damage and reduce inflammation, which are key factors in the development of chronic illnesses.

2.2 Detrimental Effects of Processed Foods

Processed foods, on the other hand, are often laden with unhealthy fats, refined sugars, artificial additives, and preservatives. These foods can have detrimental effects on health, contributing to a range of issues from obesity to chronic diseases.

Nutrient Deficiency: During the processing of foods, many essential nutrients are stripped away, leaving behind empty calories. Consuming a diet high in processed foods can lead to nutrient deficiencies, which can impair bodily functions and increase the risk of health problems.

Increased Inflammation: Processed foods often contain trans fats, refined sugars, and artificial additives that can trigger inflammation in the body. Chronic inflammation is a major contributor to a variety of health issues, including heart disease, diabetes, and autoimmune disorders.

Blood Sugar Spikes: Foods high in refined sugars and carbohydrates can cause rapid spikes in blood sugar levels, followed by crashes that can lead to fatigue, irritability, and cravings for more sugary foods. Over time, this can contribute to insulin resistance and increase the risk of type 2 diabetes.

Digestive Problems: The lack of fiber in processed foods can lead to digestive issues such as constipation and an imbalanced gut microbiome. A healthy gut is essential for overall health, as it plays a role in nutrient absorption, immune function, and even mental health.

Addiction and Overeating: Processed foods are often designed to be hyper-palatable, with combinations of sugar, fat, and salt that can be addictive and lead to overeating. This can contribute to weight gain and increase the risk of obesity-related diseases.

2.3 Foods to Embrace

Embracing a diet rich in nutrient-dense, plant-based foods is a powerful way to support your health. Here are some categories and examples of foods to include in your daily meals:

Fruits:

- **Berries:** Strawberries, blueberries, raspberries, and blackberries. These are high in antioxidants, vitamins, and fiber.

- **Citrus Fruits:** Oranges, grapefruits, lemons, and limes. Rich in vitamin C, they help boost the immune system.

- **Tropical Fruits:** Bananas, mangoes, pineapples, and papayas. These provide a variety of vitamins, minerals, and enzymes that aid digestion.

- **Apples, Pears, grapes, and melons.** These are packed with vitamins, antioxidants, and fiber.

Vegetables:

- **Leafy Greens:** Spinach, kale, arugula, and Swiss chard. Packed with vitamins A, C, and K, as well as iron and calcium.

- **Cruciferous Vegetables:** Broccoli, cauliflower, Brussels sprouts, and cabbage. Known for their cancer-fighting properties.

- **Root Vegetables:** Carrots, beets, sweet potatoes, and radishes. High in fiber and essential nutrients like potassium and magnesium.

Whole Grains:

- **Quinoa:** A complete protein source, rich in fiber, magnesium, and antioxidants.

- **Brown Rice:** Provides sustained energy and supports digestive health.

- **Oats:** High in beta-glucans, which can help lower cholesterol levels and improve heart health.

- **Barley, Farro and Millet:** provide sustained energy and are rich in fiber.

Legumes:

- **Lentils:** An excellent source of protein, fiber, iron, and folate.

- **Chickpeas:** High in protein and fiber, they support digestive health and help maintain stable blood sugar levels.

- **Black Beans:** Rich in protein, fiber, and antioxidants, supporting heart health and reducing inflammation.

- **Peas:** Excellent source of plant-based protein and fiber.

Nuts and Seeds:

- **Almonds:** Provide healthy fats, protein, and vitamin E, which is beneficial for skin health.

- **Walnuts:** High in omega-3 fatty acids, which support brain health and reduce inflammation.

- **Chia Seeds:** Packed with omega-3s, fiber, and antioxidants, they support heart health and digestion.

- **Flaxseeds, Sunflower Seeds, and Pumpkin Seeds:** offer healthy fats, protein, and essential nutrients.

Healthy Fats:

- **Avocados:** Rich in monounsaturated fats, fiber, and potassium, supporting heart health and reducing inflammation.

- **Olives:** Provide healthy fats and antioxidants, supporting heart health and reducing oxidative stress.

- **Coconut:** Contains medium-chain triglycerides (MCTs) that provide quick energy and support metabolic health.

Herbs and Spices:

- **Turmeric:** Contains curcumin, a powerful anti-inflammatory and antioxidant compound.

- **Ginger:** Supports digestion, reduces nausea, and has anti-inflammatory properties.

- **Garlic:** Known for its immune-boosting properties and ability to reduce blood pressure.

- **Cinnamon:** has anti-inflammatory and antioxidant properties.

Incorporating a variety of these foods into your diet ensures you get a wide range of nutrients, supporting overall health and vitality. By focusing on whole, unprocessed foods, you can provide your body with the essential nutrients it needs to function optimally and promote natural healing.

2.4 Foods to Avoid

While incorporating beneficial foods into your diet is essential, it is equally important to be aware of foods and substances that can negatively impact your health. Avoiding these can significantly improve your overall well-being and help you achieve optimal health.

Processed Foods: Processed foods are typically high in unhealthy fats, refined sugars, and artificial additives. These foods often contain empty calories, which contribute to weight gain without providing essential nutrients. Examples of processed foods to avoid include packaged snacks, fast food, and ready-to-eat meals. These products are often high in trans fats and hydrogenated oils, which can increase the risk of heart disease and other chronic conditions.

Refined Sugars: Refined sugars are found in many sweetened beverages, candies, baked goods, and sugary cereals. Consuming too much refined sugar can lead to blood sugar spikes and crashes, resulting in fatigue, irritability, and cravings for more sugar. Over time, excessive sugar intake can contribute to insulin resistance, obesity, and an increased risk of type 2 diabetes. To maintain stable blood sugar levels and overall health, it is best to avoid foods and drinks with high amounts of added sugars.

Refined Grains: Refined grains, such as white bread, white rice, and pasta made from refined flour, have been stripped of their nutrients and fiber during processing. This makes them less nutritious and can lead to rapid spikes in blood sugar levels. Opt for whole grains like quinoa, brown rice, and whole wheat bread to ensure you get the full nutritional benefits of grains.

Trans Fats and Hydrogenated Oils: Trans fats and hydrogenated oils are commonly found in margarine, shortening, and many processed foods. These unhealthy fats can increase LDL (bad) cholesterol levels and lower HDL (good) cholesterol levels, raising the risk of heart disease. It's important to read food labels and avoid products containing partially hydrogenated oils to protect your heart health.

Artificial Sweeteners and Additives: Artificial sweeteners like aspartame and saccharin, as well as additives like monosodium glutamate (MSG), can have adverse health effects. While they are often marketed as low-calorie alternatives, they can still contribute to health issues such as headaches, digestive problems, and metabolic disturbances. Choose natural sweeteners like honey or maple syrup in moderation and avoid products with artificial additives.

Excessive Animal Products: High consumption of red meat, processed meats, and dairy can contribute to inflammation and increase the risk of chronic diseases. Processed meats, in particular, are often high in sodium and preservatives, which can have negative health effects. To maintain a balanced diet, focus on plant-based protein sources and limit your intake of animal products. When consuming animal products, choose organic, pasture-raised options to reduce exposure to hormones and antibiotics.

High-Sodium Foods: High-sodium foods, such as canned soups, processed meats, and snack foods, can lead to high blood pressure and other health issues. Excessive sodium intake can cause fluid retention, increasing the workload on the heart and kidneys. To reduce your sodium intake, opt for fresh, whole foods and use herbs and spices to flavor your meals.

Artificial Colors and Preservatives: Many processed foods contain artificial colors and preservatives to enhance appearance and shelf life. These additives can have negative effects on health, including allergic reactions and hyperactivity in children. To avoid these harmful substances, choose fresh, whole foods and read labels carefully.

3. Hydration and Its Importance

3.1 Importance of Staying Hydrated for Overall Health

Water is essential for life and plays a critical role in maintaining every bodily function. Staying properly hydrated is fundamental to holistic health, as water is involved in digestion, nutrient absorption, circulation, and temperature regulation. Every cell, tissue, and organ in your body requires water to function optimally.

Key Functions of Water in the Body:

- **Digestion and Nutrient Absorption:** Water aids in the breakdown of food, making nutrients more accessible for absorption in the intestines. It helps dissolve minerals and nutrients, allowing them to be transported to cells where they are needed.

- **Circulation and Detoxification:** Adequate hydration ensures that blood can efficiently transport oxygen and nutrients to cells and remove waste products. Water helps flush out toxins through urine, sweat, and bowel movements, supporting the body's natural detoxification processes.

- **Temperature Regulation:** Water is crucial for regulating body temperature. Through sweating and respiration, water helps dissipate heat and maintain a stable internal temperature, preventing overheating and dehydration.

- **Joint Lubrication and Skin Health:** Water keeps joints lubricated, reducing friction and wear, which can help prevent joint pain and stiffness. It also maintains skin hydration, keeping it elastic and vibrant.

- **Cognitive Function and Energy Levels:** Dehydration can impair cognitive function, leading to difficulties in concentration, memory, and mood regulation. Proper hydration supports brain function and can improve energy levels, reducing feelings of fatigue and enhancing mental clarity.

Daily Intake Recommendations:

- **Aim for at least 8 glasses (about 2 liters) of water per day.** This is a general recommendation, but the amount of water each person needs can vary based on factors like age, gender, activity level, and climate.

- **Listen to your body:** Thirst is a natural indicator that your body needs water. Drink when you're thirsty and monitor the color of your urine—light yellow typically indicates adequate hydration.

Tips for Staying Hydrated:

- **Start Your Day with Water:** Begin your day by drinking a glass of water to rehydrate after a night's sleep. Adding a slice of lemon can enhance flavor and provide additional health benefits.

- **Carry a Water Bottle:** Keep a reusable water bottle with you throughout the day to encourage regular drinking. This can help you stay mindful of your water intake.

- **Set Reminders:** Use alarms or smartphone apps to remind you to drink water at regular intervals, especially if you tend to forget.

- **Incorporate Water-Rich Foods:** Eat fruits and vegetables with high water content, such as cucumbers, watermelon, oranges, and strawberries. These can contribute to your overall hydration.

- **Monitor Physical Activity:** Increase your water intake during and after physical activity to compensate for fluid loss through sweat. Hydrating before, during, and after exercise is crucial for performance and recovery.

- **Adjust for Climate:** In hot or humid weather, you may need to drink more water to stay hydrated. Similarly, high altitudes can increase your water needs.

3.2 Benefits of Drinking Clean Water and Its Impact on Health

The quality of the water you consume is just as important as the quantity. Drinking clean, filtered water can have a significant impact on your health, as it reduces your exposure to contaminants and supports overall well-being.

Benefits of Clean, Filtered Water:

- **Reduction of Contaminants:** Filtering water helps remove harmful substances such as chlorine, heavy metals (like lead and mercury), pesticides, and bacterial contaminants. These substances can have adverse health effects, including digestive issues, neurological problems, and increased risk of chronic diseases.

- **Improved Taste and Smell:** Clean water often tastes and smells better, making it more pleasant to drink. This can encourage you to drink more water, helping you stay hydrated.

- **Enhanced Nutrient Absorption:** Clean water supports the body's ability to absorb nutrients effectively. Contaminants in water can interfere with nutrient absorption and disrupt bodily functions.

- **Support for Detoxification:** Drinking clean water aids in the detoxification process, helping to flush out toxins and waste products from the body more efficiently. This supports liver and kidney function, which are crucial for detoxification.

- **Overall Health and Well-being:** Consuming clean water contributes to overall health by supporting all bodily functions. It helps maintain clear skin, healthy digestion, and robust immune function.

How to Ensure Clean Water:

- **Use a Water Filter:** Invest in a high-quality water filter for your home. Options include activated carbon filters, reverse osmosis systems, and water distillers. Choose a filter that effectively removes contaminants specific to your area.

- **Regular Maintenance:** If you use a filtration system, ensure it is maintained and replaced according to the manufacturer's instructions to ensure it continues to function effectively.

- **Bottled Water:** In situations where filtered water is not available, opt for bottled water from a reputable source. Be mindful of plastic waste and recycle when possible.

- **Boil Water:** In emergencies or when the quality of water is uncertain, boiling water can help kill bacteria and viruses, making it safer to drink.

Hydration is a fundamental aspect of holistic health, impacting every function of the body from digestion to cognitive performance. By understanding the critical role of hydration, adhering to daily intake recommendations, and ensuring the water you drink is clean and filtered, you can significantly enhance your overall health and well-being. Embrace these practices to support your body's natural healing abilities and maintain optimal hydration for a vibrant, healthy life.

4. Incorporating Superfoods and Antifungals

4.1 Health Benefits

Superfoods and antifungal foods are powerful allies in the journey towards optimal health. These nutrient-dense foods provide a multitude of benefits that support the body's natural healing processes, enhance immunity, and promote overall well-being.

Superfoods

Superfoods are rich in vitamins, minerals, antioxidants, and other essential nutrients. They offer a concentrated source of nutrition and have been linked to numerous health benefits, including:

- **Boosting Immune Function:** **Berries** (Blueberries, Strawberries, Raspberries) are high in vitamin C and antioxidants, help strengthen the immune system and protect against infections; **Citrus Fruits** (Oranges, Grapefruits, Lemons) are packed with vitamin C, enhance immune function and support skin health; **Leafy Greens** are high in vitamins E, which strengthen the immune system and help the body fight off infections.

- **Reducing Inflammation:** **Turmeric** Contains curcumin, a powerful anti-inflammatory compound that can help reduce inflammation and pain; **Ginger** is known for its anti-inflammatory and antioxidant properties, can help alleviate symptoms of arthritis and improve digestive health; **Fatty Fish** (Salmon, Mackerel, Sardines) is rich in omega-3 fatty acids, which reduce inflammation and support heart health.

- **Enhancing Digestive Health:** **Chia Seeds** are high in fiber, promote healthy digestion and regular bowel movements; **Flaxseeds** are rich in fiber and omega-3 fatty acids, support digestive health and reduce inflammation; **Legumes** (Lentils, Chickpeas, Black Beans) are packed with fiber, these foods support a healthy gut microbiome and improve digestion.

- **Supporting Heart Health:** **Nuts** (Almonds, Walnuts, Pecans) and **Seeds** are high in healthy fats that can lower bad cholesterol levels and reduce the risk of heart disease; **Avocados** contain monounsaturated fats that support heart health and reduce inflammation; **Dark Chocolate** is rich in flavonoids, can improve blood flow and lower blood pressure.

- **Boosting Energy Levels:** **Quinoa** is a complete protein source that provides sustained energy and supports muscle health; **Spirulina** is a blue-green algae rich in protein, vitamins, and minerals, boosts energy levels and improves endurance, and **Bananas** are high in potassium and natural sugars, provide a quick energy boost and support muscle function.

Antifungal Foods

Antifungal foods help to combat fungal infections and maintain a healthy balance of microorganisms in the body. These foods have natural properties that inhibit the growth of harmful fungi and support overall health. Key benefits include:

- **Fighting Candida:** **Garlic** contains allicin, a compound with potent antifungal properties that can help control Candida overgrowth and improve immune function; **Coconut Oil** is rich in caprylic acid and lauric acid, which have antifungal properties that can help combat Candida and other fungal infections; **Apple Cider Vinegar** contains acetic acid, which can inhibit the growth of Candida and balance the body's pH levels.

- **Supporting Immune Health:** **Leafy Greens** (Spinach, Kale, Swiss Chard) are high in vitamins A and C, boost immune function and support overall health; **Cruciferous Vegetables** (Broccoli, Cauliflower, Brussels Sprouts) contain sulfur compounds that support detoxification and enhance immune function; **Citrus Fruits** (Oranges, Lemons, Limes) provide vitamin C and antioxidants that strengthen the immune system and protect against infections.

- **Promoting Gut Health:** <u>Yogurt and Kefir</u> are rich in probiotics, these fermented foods support a healthy gut microbiome and improve digestion; <u>Fermented Vegetables</u> (Sauerkraut, Kimchi) provide beneficial bacteria that support gut health and boost immune function; <u>Asparagus</u> contains prebiotics that feed beneficial gut bacteria and support a healthy digestive system.

- **Detoxification:** <u>Leafy Greens</u> (Spinach, Kale, Arugula) are high in chlorophyll, which supports detoxification and helps remove toxins from the body; <u>Cruciferous Vegetables</u> (Broccoli, Cabbage, Brussels Sprouts) contain compounds that enhance liver detoxification and support overall health; <u>Herbs</u> (Cilantro, Parsley) help remove heavy metals and other toxins from the body, supporting detoxification and overall health.

4.2 How to Include Superfoods and Antifungals in Daily Meals

Incorporating superfoods and antifungal foods into your daily meals is easier than you might think. Here are some practical tips and delicious ideas to get you started:

Breakfast:
- **Smoothie Bowls:** Blend spinach, kale, or other leafy greens with berries, a banana, and a splash of almond milk. Top with chia seeds, flaxseeds, and a drizzle of honey for a nutrient-packed start to your day.
- **Overnight Oats:** Mix oats with chia seeds, almond milk, and a dash of cinnamon. Let it sit overnight and top with fresh berries, nuts, and a spoonful of Greek yogurt in the morning.

Lunch:
- **Quinoa Salad:** Toss cooked quinoa with chopped vegetables like bell peppers, cucumbers, and cherry tomatoes. Add avocado, chickpeas, and a sprinkle of hemp seeds. Dress with olive oil, lemon juice, and a pinch of sea salt.
- **Veggie Wraps:** Fill whole-grain wraps with hummus, sliced avocado, spinach, shredded carrots, and sprouts. Add a sprinkle of turmeric and black pepper for an extra health boost.

Dinner:
- **Stir-Fry:** Sauté a mix of vegetables such as broccoli, bell peppers, and snap peas with garlic and ginger. Add tofu or tempeh and a splash of tamari sauce. Serve over brown rice or quinoa.
- **Stuffed Sweet Potatoes:** Bake sweet potatoes and fill them with a mixture of black beans, corn, diced tomatoes, and avocado. Top with a sprinkle of nutritional yeast and fresh cilantro.

Snacks:
- **Trail Mix:** Combine a variety of nuts, seeds, and dried fruits. Add in a few pieces of dark chocolate for a delicious and energizing snack.
- **Veggie Sticks with Dip:** Slice cucumbers, carrots, and bell peppers. Serve with a dip made from blended avocado, garlic, lemon juice, and a pinch of salt.

Beverages:
- **Green Tea Latte:** Whisk matcha powder with hot water and blend with steamed almond milk. Sweeten with a touch of honey if desired.
- **Detox Water:** Infuse water with slices of lemon, cucumber, and fresh mint leaves. Let it sit for a few hours to enhance the flavors and benefits.

Incorporating Antifungal Foods:

- **Garlic:** Add minced garlic to sauces, soups, and stir-fries to boost flavor and antifungal benefits.

- **Coconut Oil:** Use coconut oil in cooking or add it to smoothies for its antifungal properties.

- **Apple Cider Vinegar:** Make a salad dressing with apple cider vinegar, olive oil, and herbs.

- **Leafy Greens:** Include a variety of leafy greens in salads, smoothies, and sides to support detoxification and gut health.

5. Using Herbs and Spices for Health

5.1 Medicinal Properties: Health Benefits of Common Herbs and Spices

Herbs and spices are not only flavor enhancers but also potent natural remedies with numerous health benefits. Incorporating them into your diet can support various aspects of your health, from boosting immunity to reducing inflammation.

Turmeric:

- **Health Benefits:** Contains curcumin, a powerful anti-inflammatory and antioxidant compound. It can help reduce inflammation, improve brain function, and lower the risk of heart disease.
- **Uses:** Turmeric can be added to curries, soups, smoothies, and teas.

Ginger:

- **Health Benefits:** Known for its anti-inflammatory and antioxidant properties, ginger can help alleviate nausea, reduce muscle pain, and improve digestion.
- **Uses:** Ginger can be used in teas, stir-fries, baked goods, and smoothies.

Garlic:

- **Health Benefits:** Rich in allicin, garlic has strong antibacterial, antiviral, and antifungal properties. It can help boost the immune system, lower blood pressure, and reduce the risk of heart disease.
- **Uses:** Garlic can be added to sauces, soups, marinades, and roasted vegetables.

Cinnamon:

- **Health Benefits:** Contains cinnamaldehyde, which has anti-inflammatory and antioxidant effects. Cinnamon can help regulate blood sugar levels, reduce heart disease risk, and improve metabolic health.
- **Uses:** Cinnamon can be sprinkled on oatmeal, added to baked goods, and incorporated into teas and smoothies.

Peppermint:

- **Health Benefits:** Contains menthol, which has soothing and cooling properties. Peppermint can help relieve digestive issues, reduce headaches, and improve respiratory function.
- **Uses:** Peppermint can be used in teas, desserts, and as a flavoring for water.

Basil:

- **Health Benefits:** Rich in essential oils and antioxidants, basil can help reduce inflammation, support cardiovascular health, and improve digestion.
- **Uses:** Basil can be added to salads, pasta dishes, and pesto.

Rosemary:

- **Health Benefits:** Contains rosmarinic acid, which has anti-inflammatory and antioxidant properties. Rosemary can help improve digestion, enhance memory, and reduce oxidative stress.
- **Uses:** Rosemary can be used in marinades, roasted vegetables, and soups.

Oregano:

- **Health Benefits:** High in antioxidants and antibacterial compounds, oregano can help boost the immune system, improve digestion, and fight off infections.
- **Uses:** Oregano can be added to sauces, salads, and meat dishes.

Cayenne Pepper:

- **Health Benefits:** Contains capsaicin, which has pain-relieving properties and can help boost metabolism, reduce hunger, and improve digestive health.
- **Uses:** Cayenne pepper can be used in spicy dishes, soups, and as a seasoning for meats and vegetables.

Parsley:

- **Health Benefits:** Rich in vitamins A, C, and K, parsley can help support bone health and boost the immune system.
- **Uses:** Parsley can be added to salads, soups, and as a garnish for various dishes.

5.2 Practical Tips for Adding Herbs and Spices to Meals

Incorporating herbs and spices into your meals can be simple and enjoyable. Here are some practical tips to help you get started:

- **Start Small**: Begin by adding small amounts of herbs and spices to your dishes and gradually increase the quantity as you become accustomed to their flavors.

- **Experiment with Combinations**: Mix and match different herbs and spices to find combinations that you enjoy. For example, basil and oregano pair well in Italian dishes, while ginger and turmeric complement each other in Asian cuisine.

- **Use Fresh and Dried Forms**: Both fresh and dried herbs and spices have their place in cooking. Fresh herbs are great for salads, garnishes, and light dishes, while dried herbs and spices are ideal for soups, stews, and marinades.

- **Infuse Oils and Vinegars**: Create flavored oils and vinegars by infusing them with herbs and spices. This can add a unique twist to your salads and cooking.

- **Incorporate into Drinks**: Add herbs and spices to your beverages for an extra health boost. Try adding ginger to your tea, mint to your water, or cinnamon to your coffee.

- **Enhance Your Baking**: Spices like cinnamon, nutmeg, and ginger can add warmth and depth to baked goods. Experiment with adding these spices to your cookies, cakes, and breads.

- **Make Herbal Teas**: Create your own herbal teas by steeping fresh or dried herbs in hot water. This is a great way to enjoy the health benefits of herbs like peppermint, chamomile, and rosemary.

- **Use as Garnishes**: Fresh herbs like parsley, cilantro, and chives make excellent garnishes for soups, stews, and main dishes, adding a burst of flavor and color.

6. Combating Ailments with Specific Nutrients

A well-balanced diet rich in specific nutrients can significantly impact your health and help address common health issues. Here, we explore key nutrients and their roles in supporting heart health, immune function, digestive health, bone health, mental health, and overall well-being.

6.1 Heart Health

Omega-3 Fatty Acids:
- **Benefits**: Omega-3 fatty acids, found in fatty fish (salmon, mackerel, sardines), flaxseeds, and walnuts, play a crucial role in heart health. They help reduce inflammation, lower blood pressure, decrease triglyceride levels, and reduce the risk of arrhythmias (irregular heartbeats).
- **How to Incorporate**: Aim to eat fatty fish at least twice a week, sprinkle ground flaxseeds on your oatmeal or yogurt, and snack on a handful of walnuts.

Fiber:
- **Benefits**: Dietary fiber, found in whole grains, fruits, vegetables, and legumes, helps reduce cholesterol levels, control blood sugar levels, and maintain a healthy weight—all of which are beneficial for heart health.
- **How to Incorporate**: Include a variety of fiber-rich foods in your diet, such as oats, berries, beans, and leafy greens. Aim for at least 25-30 grams of fiber per day.

Antioxidants (Vitamin C and E):
- **Benefits**: Antioxidants like vitamin C and vitamin E help protect the heart by neutralizing free radicals, reducing oxidative stress, and preventing the buildup of plaque in the arteries. Sources include citrus fruits, berries, nuts, seeds, and green leafy vegetables.
- **How to Incorporate**: Eat a variety of colorful fruits and vegetables daily, include nuts and seeds in your meals.

6.2 Immune Support

Vitamin C:

- **Benefits:** Vitamin C is a powerful antioxidant that enhances the immune system by stimulating the production of white blood cells, which help fight infections. It also helps the body absorb iron from plant-based foods.
- **Sources:** Citrus fruits (oranges, grapefruits, lemons), strawberries, bell peppers, broccoli, and kiwi.
- **How to Incorporate:** Add a variety of vitamin C-rich fruits and vegetables to your meals. A daily intake of 75-90 mg is recommended.

Vitamin D:

- **Benefits:** Vitamin D is essential for immune function, as it helps regulate the immune response and enhances the pathogen-fighting effects of monocytes and macrophages. It also plays a role in reducing inflammation.
- **Sources:** Sun exposure, fatty fish, fortified dairy products, and egg yolks.
- **How to Incorporate:** Spend time outdoors in sunlight, consume vitamin D-rich foods, and consider a supplement if necessary (consult with a healthcare provider).

Zinc:

- **Benefits:** Zinc is crucial for immune cell development and communication and plays a role in inflammatory response. It is also essential for wound healing.
- **Sources:** Shellfish, meat, legumes, seeds, nuts, and whole grains.
- **How to Incorporate:** Include a variety of zinc-rich foods in your diet, such as pumpkin seeds, chickpeas, and quinoa.

6.3 Digestive Health

Probiotics:

- **Benefits:** Probiotics are beneficial bacteria that support a healthy gut microbiome, enhance digestion, and boost the immune system. They help balance the gut flora and prevent gastrointestinal issues such as bloating, gas, and constipation.
- **Sources:** Yogurt, kefir, sauerkraut, kimchi, miso, and kombucha.
- **How to Incorporate:** Include fermented foods in your daily diet, such as a serving of yogurt with breakfast or a side of sauerkraut with lunch or dinner.

Fiber:

- **Benefits:** Fiber is essential for digestive health as it adds bulk to the stool, aiding in regular bowel movements and preventing constipation. It also feeds the beneficial bacteria in the gut, promoting a healthy microbiome.
- **Sources:** Whole grains, fruits, vegetables, legumes, nuts, and seeds.
- **How to Incorporate:** Ensure your diet includes a variety of fiber-rich foods, aiming for at least 25-30 grams per day. Add beans to salads, snack on fruits and nuts, and choose whole grains over refined grains.

Water:

- **Benefits:** Staying hydrated is crucial for digestive health, as water helps break down food, absorb nutrients, and maintain regular bowel movements.
- **Sources:** Water, herbal teas, and water-rich fruits and vegetables (cucumbers, watermelon, oranges).
- **How to Incorporate:** Drink plenty of water throughout the day and include water-rich foods in your diet.

6.4 Bone Health

Calcium:
- **Benefits:** Calcium is essential for building and maintaining strong bones and teeth. It also plays a crucial role in muscle function, nerve transmission, and blood clotting.
- **Sources:** Dairy products (milk, cheese, yogurt), leafy greens (kale, broccoli), almonds, and fortified plant-based milks.
- **How to Incorporate:** Include calcium-rich foods in your diet, such as a serving of yogurt for breakfast, a kale salad for lunch, and almond milk in your smoothie.

Vitamin D:
- **Benefits:** Vitamin D enhances calcium absorption in the gut and maintains adequate serum calcium and phosphate concentrations, which are necessary for bone formation and remodeling.
- **Sources:** Sun exposure, fatty fish, fortified dairy products, and egg yolks.
- **How to Incorporate:** Spend time outdoors in sunlight, consume vitamin D-rich foods, and consider a supplement if necessary (consult with a healthcare provider).

Magnesium:
- **Benefits:** Magnesium is involved in bone formation and influences the activities of osteoblasts and osteoclasts. It also plays a role in converting vitamin D into its active form, which aids in calcium absorption.
- **Sources:** Nuts, seeds, whole grains, green leafy vegetables, and legumes.
- **How to Incorporate:** Add magnesium-rich foods to your diet, such as a handful of almonds, a serving of spinach, or a portion of brown rice.

6.5 Mental Health

Omega-3 Fatty Acids:
- **Benefits:** Omega-3 fatty acids, particularly EPA and DHA, are crucial for brain health. They support cognitive function, reduce symptoms of depression and anxiety, and protect against neurodegenerative diseases.
- **Sources:** Fatty fish (salmon, mackerel, sardines), flaxseeds, chia seeds, and walnuts.
- **How to Incorporate:** Aim to eat fatty fish at least twice a week, add chia seeds to your smoothies, and snack on walnuts.

B Vitamins:
- **Benefits:** B vitamins, especially B6, B9 (folate), and B12, are essential for brain health. They help produce neurotransmitters like serotonin, dopamine, and GABA, which regulate mood and cognitive function.
- **Sources:** Whole grains, leafy greens, legumes, eggs, and lean meats.
- **How to Incorporate:** Include a variety of B vitamin-rich foods in your diet, such as a serving of beans, a spinach salad, or a portion of lean chicken.

Antioxidants:
- **Benefits:** Antioxidants, such as vitamins C and E, protect brain cells from oxidative stress and inflammation, which can impair cognitive function and contribute to mental health disorders.
- **Sources:** Berries, citrus fruits, nuts, seeds, and green leafy vegetables.
- **How to Incorporate:** Eat a variety of colorful fruits and vegetables daily, and include nuts and seeds in your meals and snacks.

Understanding the role of specific nutrients in combating common health issues is essential for maintaining optimal health. By incorporating these key nutrients into your diet, you can support heart health, enhance immune function, promote digestive well-being, strengthen bones, and improve mental health. Remember, a varied and balanced diet, rich in whole, unprocessed foods, is the best way to ensure you get all the nutrients your body needs to thrive.

7. Significance of Organic and Non-GMO Foods

7.1 Benefits of Organic Foods: Nutritional and Health Advantages of Organic Produce

Choosing organic foods can have a significant positive impact on your health and well-being. Organic farming practices aim to produce food without the use of synthetic pesticides, herbicides, fertilizers, and genetically modified organisms (GMOs). Here are some key benefits of consuming organic produce:

Higher Nutrient Content:

- **Vitamins and Minerals:** Studies have shown that organic fruits and vegetables can have higher levels of vitamins and minerals compared to conventionally grown produce. For instance, organic tomatoes and strawberries have been found to contain more vitamin C and antioxidants.

- **Antioxidants:** Organic produce often has higher concentrations of antioxidants, such as flavonoids and carotenoids, which help protect the body from oxidative stress and inflammation. Antioxidants play a crucial role in preventing chronic diseases like heart disease and cancer.

Reduced Exposure to Pesticides and Chemicals:

- **Health Risks of Pesticides:** Conventional farming uses synthetic pesticides and herbicides, which can leave residues on food. Long-term exposure to these chemicals has been linked to various health issues, including hormone disruption, neurological problems, and an increased risk of cancer.

- **Cleaner Food:** Organic farming avoids the use of synthetic chemicals, reducing your exposure to potentially harmful substances. This is particularly important for vulnerable populations, such as pregnant women and children, who are more susceptible to the adverse effects of pesticides.

Better for the Environment:

- **Soil Health:** Organic farming practices, such as crop rotation, composting, and the use of natural fertilizers, help improve soil health and fertility. Healthy soil retains more nutrients and water, leading to more nutritious crops.

- **Biodiversity:** Organic farms support greater biodiversity by creating a healthier ecosystem for plants, animals, and beneficial insects. This biodiversity helps maintain balance in the environment and reduces the need for chemical interventions.

- **Water Quality:** By avoiding synthetic fertilizers and pesticides, organic farming reduces the risk of water contamination. This helps protect water sources from pollution and supports overall environmental health.

Supports Animal Welfare:

- **Ethical Practices:** Organic farming standards often include guidelines for the ethical treatment of animals, ensuring they are raised in humane conditions with access to outdoor spaces and a natural diet.

- **Healthier Animal Products:** Animals raised organically are not given antibiotics or synthetic hormones, which can end up in the food supply. As a result, organic meat, dairy, and eggs are free from these substances, making them a healthier choice.

7.2 Understanding Non-GMO Foods: Importance of Choosing Non-GMO Foods and Their Impact on Health

Genetically modified organisms (GMOs) are organisms whose genetic material has been altered using genetic engineering techniques. While GMOs are widely used in agriculture, there is growing concern about their long-term impact on health and the environment. Here's why choosing non-GMO foods is important:

Health Concerns:

- **Allergies:** Some studies suggest that GMOs may introduce new allergens into the food supply, increasing the risk of allergic reactions. Choosing non-GMO foods can help minimize this risk.

- **Antibiotic Resistance:** Certain GMOs are engineered to be resistant to antibiotics. Consuming these foods may contribute to antibiotic resistance, making it harder to treat bacterial infections.

- **Unknown Long-Term Effects:** The long-term health effects of consuming GMOs are not yet fully understood. By choosing non-GMO foods, you reduce your exposure to these potential risks.

Environmental Impact:

- **Biodiversity Loss:** GMO crops are often engineered for uniformity, which can lead to a reduction in crop diversity. This loss of biodiversity makes ecosystems more vulnerable to pests, diseases, and changing climate conditions.

- **Chemical Use:** Many GMO crops are designed to be resistant to herbicides, leading to increased herbicide use. This can result in environmental contamination, harm to wildlife, and the development of herbicide-resistant weeds.

Support for Sustainable Agriculture:

- **Organic and Non-GMO Synergy:** Organic farming practices exclude the use of GMOs. By choosing organic and non-GMO foods, you support sustainable agriculture that prioritizes environmental health, animal welfare, and food safety.

- **Consumer Demand:** Choosing non-GMO foods sends a message to producers and policymakers about the importance of sustainable and transparent food production practices.

Choosing organic and non-GMO foods offers numerous benefits for your health and the environment. Organic produce is often richer in nutrients and free from harmful pesticides, while non-GMO foods help avoid potential health risks and support biodiversity. By making informed choices about the foods you consume, you can contribute to a healthier lifestyle and a more sustainable world.

8. Balanced pH: Alkaline vs. Acidic Foods

8.1 Understanding Body pH: Explanation of Body pH and Its Significance

The concept of pH (potential of Hydrogen) measures the acidity or alkalinity of a substance on a scale from 0 to 14, with 7 being neutral. A pH below 7 is acidic, and above 7 is alkaline. The body maintains a tightly regulated pH level, with blood typically ranging between 7.35 and 7.45, which is slightly alkaline.

Maintaining this pH balance is crucial for various bodily functions, including:

- **Enzyme Function:** Many enzymes that drive biochemical reactions in the body function optimally within a narrow pH range.

- **Metabolic Processes:** Proper pH levels are essential for metabolism, including the production of energy.

- **Oxygen Transport:** Hemoglobin in the blood carries oxygen more efficiently at the optimal pH level.

- **Electrolyte Balance:** pH balance helps regulate the body's electrolytes, including sodium, potassium, and calcium, which are crucial for nerve function, muscle contraction, and hydration.

When the body's pH levels become too acidic or too alkaline, it can disrupt these processes and lead to various health issues. An overly acidic environment can result in decreased bone density, muscle loss, and an increased risk of chronic diseases. Conversely, excessive alkalinity, although rare, can lead to conditions such as metabolic alkalosis.

8.2 Benefits of an Alkaline Diet and How to Balance pH Through Food Choices

Diet plays a significant role in maintaining the body's pH balance. Foods can be classified as either acid-forming or alkaline-forming based on their effect on the body's pH after digestion and metabolism, not their initial pH.

Alkaline-Forming Foods: These foods help promote a more alkaline environment in the body, which can support overall health. Some benefits of an alkaline diet include improved bone health, enhanced muscle function, and reduced inflammation.

- **Fruits:** Apples, bananas, berries, citrus fruits, grapes, melons.

  Benefits: High in vitamins, minerals, and antioxidants that support immune function and reduce oxidative stress.

- **Vegetables:** Leafy greens (spinach, kale, arugula), broccoli, cucumbers, carrots, sweet potatoes.

  Benefits: Rich in fiber, vitamins, and minerals that aid digestion and provide essential nutrients.

- **Nuts and Seeds:** Almonds, chia seeds, flaxseeds.

  Benefits: Provide healthy fats, protein, and fiber that support heart health and digestion.

- **Legumes:** Lentils, chickpeas, black beans.

  Benefits: High in protein and fiber, helping maintain stable blood sugar levels and supporting gut health.

- **Herbs and Spices:** Garlic, ginger, turmeric.

  Benefits: Contain anti-inflammatory and antioxidant properties that enhance overall health.

Acid-Forming Foods: These foods can contribute to an acidic environment in the body when consumed in excess. While not all acidic foods are harmful, it's essential to balance them with alkaline foods to maintain optimal health.

- **Animal Products:** Meat, poultry, fish, eggs.

  Insights: Provide essential proteins and nutrients but should be balanced with plant-based foods.

- **Dairy Products:** Cheese, milk, yogurt.

  Insights: Good sources of calcium and protein, but can be acidic-forming.

- **Grains:** Wheat, rice, oats.

  Insights: Provide essential carbohydrates and fiber but can be acid-forming, especially refined grains.

- **Processed Foods:** Fast food, snacks, sugary drinks.

  Insights: Limited nutritional value and can contribute to acidity and inflammation.

Tips for Balancing pH Through Food Choices:

- **Increase Intake of Alkaline Foods:** Fill half your plate with fruits and vegetables at each meal. Incorporate a variety of colors to ensure a broad range of nutrients. Snack on raw vegetables, nuts, and seeds instead of processed snacks.

- **Limit Acid-Forming Foods:** Reduce consumption of red meat and processed foods. Opt for plant-based protein sources like legumes and nuts. Choose whole grains over refined grains to minimize acid load.

- **Stay Hydrated:** Drink plenty of water throughout the day. Adding a slice of lemon or a splash of apple cider vinegar can help alkalize your water. Herbal teas, such as chamomile or green tea, can also support pH balance.

- **Incorporate Alkaline-Rich Recipes:** Smoothies with leafy greens, fruits, and seeds make a nutrient-dense, alkaline-rich start to your day. Salads with a variety of vegetables, topped with nuts and seeds, and dressed with olive oil and lemon juice provide a balanced, alkaline meal.

- **Mindful Eating Practices:** Chew food thoroughly to aid digestion and nutrient absorption. Practice portion control and balance meals with a mix of alkaline and acid-forming foods.

Maintaining a balanced pH through diet is an essential aspect of holistic health. By incorporating more alkaline-forming foods and reducing the intake of acid-forming foods, you can support your body's natural pH balance, enhance metabolic processes, and improve overall well-being. Remember, the key is balance and variety in your diet, ensuring that you provide your body with the nutrients it needs to thrive.

9. Practical Tips for a Healthful Dietary Regimen

9.1 How to Structure Meals Throughout the Day

Establishing a consistent daily eating pattern can help regulate your metabolism, maintain energy levels, and support overall health. Here are some guidelines for structuring your meals throughout the day:

Breakfast:

- **Importance:** Breakfast kick-starts your metabolism and provides the energy needed to begin your day. It can help improve concentration and performance.

- **Recommendations:** Aim for a balanced breakfast that includes protein, healthy fats, and complex carbohydrates. For example, a smoothie with spinach, berries, chia seeds, and almond milk, or whole-grain toast with avocado and a poached egg.

Mid-Morning Snack:

- **Importance:** A healthy snack can help maintain energy levels and prevent overeating at lunch.

- **Recommendations:** Opt for a small portion of nuts, a piece of fruit, or yogurt with a sprinkle of granola.

Lunch:

- **Importance:** A nutritious lunch provides the necessary fuel to sustain energy levels throughout the afternoon.

- **Recommendations:** Include a variety of vegetables, lean proteins, and whole grains. A quinoa salad with mixed vegetables and chickpeas, or a vegetable stir-fry with tofu and brown rice are great options.

Afternoon Snack:

- **Importance:** Another healthy snack can help curb cravings and keep you energized until dinner.

- **Recommendations:** Choose snacks that combine protein and fiber, such as hummus with carrot sticks, or an apple with almond butter.

Dinner:

- **Importance:** Dinner should be nourishing but not too heavy, as eating large meals late in the evening can disrupt sleep.

- **Recommendations:** Focus on vegetables, lean proteins, and healthy fats. A baked salmon fillet with a side of steamed broccoli and quinoa, or a hearty vegetable soup with a side salad are excellent choices.

Hydration:

- **Importance:** Staying hydrated throughout the day is crucial for overall health and optimal bodily function.

- **Recommendations:** Drink plenty of water, herbal teas, and eat water-rich foods like cucumbers and melons. Aim for at least 8 glasses of water per day.

9.2 Practices for Detoxifying the Body Naturally

Detoxification is the body's natural process of eliminating toxins. Supporting this process with specific practices can enhance your overall health.

Hydration:

- **Importance:** Drinking enough water helps flush toxins out of the body through urine and sweat.
- **Practice:** Start your day with a glass of warm lemon water to stimulate digestion and detoxification.

Fiber-Rich Foods:

- **Importance:** Fiber aids in the removal of waste products and supports digestive health.
- **Practice:** Incorporate plenty of fruits, vegetables, whole grains, and legumes into your diet.

Herbal Teas:

- **Importance:** Certain herbs can support liver function and detoxification.
- **Practice:** Drink herbal teas such as dandelion root, milk thistle, and green tea to support the detox process.

Sweating:

- **Importance:** Sweating helps eliminate toxins through the skin.
- **Practice:** Engage in regular physical activity, such as jogging, yoga, or using a sauna to promote sweating.

Reduce Intake of Toxins:

- **Importance:** Minimizing exposure to toxins helps the body's natural detoxification processes.
- **Practice:** Avoid processed foods, alcohol, caffeine, and reduce exposure to environmental toxins such as cigarette smoke and pollution.

Fasting:

- **Importance:** Intermittent fasting can give the digestive system a break and support detoxification.
- **Practice:** Consider incorporating intermittent fasting, such as the 16/8 method, where you fast for 16 hours and eat during an 8-hour window.

9.3 Practical Advice for Embracing a Plant-Based, Holistic Diet

Transitioning to a plant-based, holistic diet can seem daunting, but with practical steps, it becomes manageable and rewarding.

Start Gradually:

- **Importance:** Making small, incremental changes can help you adjust to a new diet without feeling overwhelmed.
- **Practice:** Begin by incorporating one plant-based meal per day and gradually increase the frequency.

Focus on Whole Foods:

- **Importance:** Whole foods are nutrient-dense and free from artificial additives.
- **Practice:** Prioritize fruits, vegetables, whole grains, legumes, nuts, and seeds. Avoid processed foods and refined sugars.

Plan Your Meals:

- **Importance:** Planning helps ensure a balanced diet and prevents reliance on convenience foods.
- **Practice:** Create a weekly meal plan and grocery list. Prepare meals in advance to save time and reduce stress.

Experiment with New Recipes:

- **Importance:** Trying new recipes keeps meals exciting and varied.
- **Practice:** Explore different cuisines and cooking methods. Join online communities or subscribe to plant-based cooking channels for inspiration.

Educate Yourself:

- **Importance:** Understanding the benefits of a plant-based diet reinforces healthy choices.
- **Practice:** Read books, watch documentaries, and follow credible sources about plant-based nutrition and holistic health.

Listen to Your Body:

- **Importance:** Everyone's nutritional needs are different. Pay attention to how different foods make you feel.
- **Practice:** Keep a food journal to track what you eat and how it affects your energy levels, digestion, and overall well-being.

Seek Support:

- **Importance:** Having a support system can make the transition smoother and more enjoyable.
- **Practice:** Connect with friends, family, or online communities who share similar health goals. Consider consulting a nutritionist or dietitian for personalized advice.

Embracing a healthful dietary regimen involves thoughtful planning and a commitment to making nutritious choices. By structuring your meals, supporting natural detoxification, and integrating the foundations of a plant-based, holistic diet, you can enhance your overall well-being and achieve optimal health. Remember, the journey to better health is a gradual process, and every positive change you make brings you one step closer to your wellness goals.

SCAN THE QR CODE:

SCAN ME

or copy and paste the url:

https://o2o.to/i/db5cYl

Section II: The Cookbook

How the Recipes Support Natural Healing

Embark on a transformative journey with recipes designed to nourish and heal your body naturally. This collection is crafted to align with Barbara O'Neill's holistic health principles, focusing on nutrient-dense, plant-based ingredients that enhance your vitality and support your body's innate healing processes.

Starting your day with energizing breakfasts, you'll find a variety of options to kickstart your metabolism and provide sustained energy. Mid-morning snacks offer nutritious boosts to keep you going until lunch, where you'll enjoy balanced, satisfying meals that provide essential vitamins, minerals, and antioxidants.

Afternoon snacks are designed to keep you fueled and satisfied, helping you avoid energy slumps and cravings. For dinner, you'll discover hearty, delicious meals that promote sustained energy and overall well-being, crafted to ensure a balance of macronutrients and micronutrients.

Special diets are also catered for, with recipes tailored to specific dietary needs such as gluten-free, keto, and paleo options, ensuring that everyone can enjoy the benefits of wholesome, healing foods. The healing and detox chapter offers powerful recipes designed to cleanse and rejuvenate your body, promoting optimal health and vitality.

By following these recipes, you'll not only enjoy a variety of delicious meals but also support your body's natural healing processes. These dishes are designed to enhance immune function, improve digestion, and provide the nutrients necessary for overall well-being. Dive in and discover how these wholesome, healing recipes can transform your diet and help you thrive naturally.

1. BREAKFAST

BLUEBERRY OAT PANCAKES

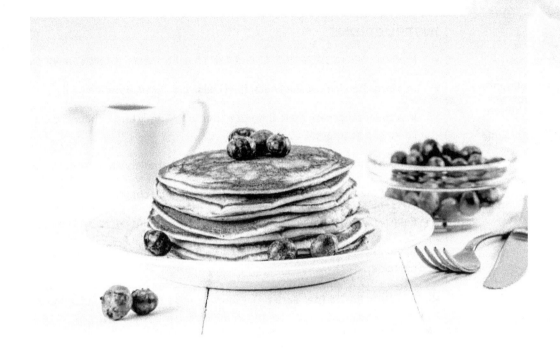

Fluffy and nutritious pancakes packed with the goodness of oats and bursting with fresh blueberries.

INGREDIENTS:	PREP TIME: 10 min	COOK TIME: 15 min	SERVINGS: 2 Servings

INGREDIENTS:	INSTRUCTIONS:
1/2 cup rolled oats 1/2 cup whole wheat flour 1 tsp baking powder 1/2 tsp baking soda 1/4 tsp salt 1 Tbsp ground flaxseed 1 cup almond milk 1 egg (or flax egg for vegan option) 1 Tbsp maple syrup 1/2 tsp vanilla extract 1/2 cup fresh blueberries 1 Tbsp coconut oil (for cooking)	• In a bowl, mix rolled oats, whole wheat flour, baking powder, baking soda, salt, and ground flaxseed. • In another bowl, whisk together almond milk, egg, maple syrup, and vanilla extract. • Combine wet and dry ingredients, stirring until just mixed. Fold in the blueberries. • Heat coconut oil in a non-stick skillet over medium heat. • Pour batter onto the skillet to form pancakes, cooking for 2-3 minutes on each side until golden brown. • Serve warm with extra blueberries and a drizzle of maple syrup if desired. **NUTRITIONAL FACTS (per Serving):** Calories: 320 | Total Fat: 10g | Saturated Fat: 2g | Fiber: 7g | Protein: 8g | Carbohydrate: 45g of which sugars: 10g | Calcium: 20% DV | Iron: 15% DV | Vitamin C: 6% DV

FLAXSEED AND ALMOND GRANOLA

A crunchy and nutritious granola, perfect for a healthy breakfast or snack, packed with the goodness of flaxseeds and almonds.

INGREDIENTS:	PREP TIME: 10 min	COOK TIME: 20 min	SERVINGS: 2 Servings
1 cup rolled oats 1/4 cup flaxseeds 1/4 cup sliced almonds 2 Tbsp almond butter 2 Tbsp honey or maple syrup 1/2 tsp vanilla extract 1/4 tsp ground cinnamon 1/4 cup dried cranberries (optional)	**INSTRUCTIONS:** • Preheat oven to 325°F (165°C) and line a baking sheet with parchment paper. • In a large bowl, mix rolled oats, flaxseeds, and sliced almonds. • In a small saucepan, melt almond butter with honey and vanilla extract over low heat, stirring until smooth. • Pour the almond butter mixture over the dry ingredients and mix until well combined. • Spread the mixture evenly on the prepared baking sheet. • Bake for 15-20 minutes, stirring halfway through, until golden brown. • Allow to cool completely before adding dried cranberries, if using. Store in an airtight container.		
NUTRITIONAL FACTS (per Serving): Calories: 280 | Total Fat: 12g | Saturated Fat: 1g | Fiber: 6g | Protein: 6g | Carbohydrate: 36g of which sugars: 12g | Iron: 10% DV | Calcium: 8% DV | Vitamin E: 20% DV			

AVOCADO AND SPINACH SMOOTHIE

A creamy and refreshing smoothie loaded with healthy fats, vitamins, and minerals to kickstart your day.

INGREDIENTS:	PREP TIME: 5 min	COOK TIME: 0 min	SERVINGS: 2 Servings
1 ripe avocado 1 cup spinach 1 banana 1 cup almond milk 1 Tbsp chia seeds 1 tsp honey (optional) 1/2 cup ice cubes	**INSTRUCTIONS:** • Combine avocado, spinach, banana, almond milk, chia seeds, honey (if using), and ice cubes in a blender. • Blend until smooth and creamy. • Pour into two glasses and serve immediately.		
NUTRITIONAL FACTS (per Serving): Calories: 280 | Total Fat: 17g | Saturated Fat: 2.5g | Fiber: 10g | Protein: 4g | Carbohydrate: 30g of which sugars: 12g | Vitamin A: 35% DV | Vitamin C: 20% DV | Calcium: 20% DV | Iron: 10% DV			

VEGAN SCRAMBLED TOFU WITH VEGETABLES

A savory and protein-packed breakfast that's perfect for starting your day with a healthy boost.

INGREDIENTS:	PREP TIME: 10 min	COOK TIME: 10 min	SERVINGS: 2 Servings

INGREDIENTS	INSTRUCTIONS / NUTRITION
1 block (14 oz) firm tofu, drained and crumbled 1 Tbsp olive oil 1/2 red bell pepper, diced 1/2 green bell pepper, diced 1 small red onion, chopped 1 cup spinach leaves, chopped 1/2 tsp turmeric powder 1/2 tsp ground cumin Salt and pepper to taste 1/4 cup nutritional yeast (optional) Fresh parsley for garnish	**INSTRUCTIONS:** • Heat olive oil in a skillet over medium heat. • Add the red and green bell peppers, and red onion. Sauté until softened, about 5 minutes. • Add crumbled tofu to the skillet, stirring to combine with the vegetables. • Season with turmeric, cumin, salt, and pepper. Cook for 3-5 minutes until the tofu is heated through and well mixed with the spices. • Stir in the chopped spinach and cook until wilted, about 2 minutes. • If using, sprinkle nutritional yeast over the scramble and mix well. • Garnish with fresh parsley and serve warm. **NUTRITIONAL FACTS (per Serving):** Calories: 180 | Total Fat: 11g | Saturated Fat: 1.5g | Fiber: 4g | Protein: 15g | Carbohydrate: 10g of which sugars: 3g | Calcium: 20% DV | Iron: 15% DV | Vitamin C: 70% DV

GREEN POWER SMOOTHIE BOWL

A vibrant and nutritious start to your day, packed with leafy greens and superfoods for an energy boost.

INGREDIENTS:	PREP TIME: 10 min	COOK TIME: 0 min	SERVINGS: 2 Servings

INGREDIENTS	INSTRUCTIONS / NUTRITION
1 cup spinach 1 frozen banana 1/2 avocado 1/2 cup almond milk 1 Tbsp chia seeds 1 Tbsp almond butter 1/2 cup mixed berries (for topping) 1 Tbsp granola (for topping) 1 tsp honey (optional, for topping)	**INSTRUCTIONS:** • Blend spinach, banana, avocado, almond milk, chia seeds, and almond butter until smooth. • Pour the smoothie into a bowl. • Top with mixed berries, granola, and honey if desired. **NUTRITIONAL FACTS (per Serving):** Calories: 350 | Total Fat: 18g | Saturated Fat: 2.5g | Fiber: 11g | Protein: 7g | Carbohydrate: 44g of which sugars: 19g | Vitamin A: 60% DV | Vitamin C: 35% DV | Calcium: 15% DV | Iron: 20% DV

QUINOA AND BERRY BREAKFAST PORRIDGE

A hearty and delicious porridge combining the goodness of quinoa and the natural sweetness of berries.

INGREDIENTS:	PREP TIME: 5 min	COOK TIME: 20 min	SERVINGS: 2 Servings
1/2 cup quinoa, rinsed 1 cup almond milk 1/2 cup water 1/2 teaspoon cinnamon 1 tablespoon maple syrup 1/2 cup mixed berries (blueberries, raspberries, strawberries) 1 tablespoon chopped almonds (for topping) 1 tablespoon chia seeds (for topping)	**INSTRUCTIONS:** • In a saucepan, combine quinoa, almond milk, water, and cinnamon. Bring to a boil. • Reduce heat and simmer for 15 minutes or until quinoa is tender. • Stir in maple syrup and half of the mixed berries. • Serve in bowls, topped with remaining berries, chopped almonds, and chia seeds.		
	NUTRITIONAL FACTS (per Serving): Calories: 310 | Total Fat: 10g | Saturated Fat: 1g | Fiber: 8g | Protein: 8g | Carbohydrate: 48g of which sugars: 12g | Vitamin C: 30% DV | Calcium: 20% DV | Iron: 15% DV		

ALMOND BUTTER BANANA TOAST

A quick and nutritious breakfast that combines the creamy richness of almond butter with the natural sweetness of banana.

INGREDIENTS:	PREP TIME: 5 min	COOK TIME: 2 min	SERVINGS: 2 Servings
2 slices whole grain bread 2 Tbsp almond butter 1 banana, sliced 1 tsp chia seeds 1/2 tsp ground cinnamon	**INSTRUCTIONS:** • Toast the whole grain bread slices until golden brown. • Spread 1 Tbsp of almond butter on each slice of toast. • Top with banana slices. • Sprinkle chia seeds and ground cinnamon over the banana slices. • Serve immediately.		
	NUTRITIONAL FACTS (per Serving): Calories: 250 | Total Fat: 12g | Saturated Fat: 1g | Fiber: 6g | Protein: 6g | Carbohydrate: 32g of which sugars: 10g | Calcium: 8% DV | Iron: 10% DV | Potassium: 12% DV		

CHIA SEED PUDDING WITH FRESH BERRIES

A delightful, nutrient-packed breakfast that's easy to prepare and perfect for busy mornings.

INGREDIENTS:	PREP TIME: 10 min	COOK TIME: 0 min	SERVINGS: 2 Servings

INGREDIENTS:	INSTRUCTIONS:
1/4 cup chia seeds 1 cup almond milk 1 Tbsp maple syrup 1/2 tsp vanilla extract 1/2 cup fresh mixed berries (strawberries, blueberries, raspberries) 1 Tbsp chopped nuts (optional, for topping)	• In a bowl, whisk together chia seeds, almond milk, maple syrup, and vanilla extract. • Cover and refrigerate overnight or for at least 4 hours until the mixture thickens. • Stir well before serving and divide into two bowls. • Top with fresh berries and chopped nuts if desired.
	NUTRITIONAL FACTS (per Serving): Calories: 230 | Total Fat: 12g | Saturated Fat: 1g | Fiber: 10g | Protein: 5g | Carbohydrate: 25g of which sugars: 12g | Calcium: 25% DV | Iron: 10% DV | Vitamin C: 20% DV

SWEET POTATO AND BLACK BEAN BREAKFAST BURRITO

A hearty and flavorful burrito that combines sweet potatoes and black beans for a nutritious start to your day.

INGREDIENTS:	PREP TIME: 15 min	COOK TIME: 20 min	SERVINGS: 2 Servings

INGREDIENTS:	INSTRUCTIONS:
1 medium sweet potato, peeled and diced 1 Tbsp olive oil 1/2 cup black beans, cooked and drained 1/2 red bell pepper, diced 1 small red onion, diced 1 tsp ground cumin 1/2 tsp smoked paprika Salt and pepper to taste 2 large whole wheat tortillas 1/4 cup fresh salsa 1 avocado, sliced Fresh cilantro for garnish	• Preheat oven to 400°F (200°C). Toss the diced sweet potato with 1/2 Tbsp olive oil, cumin, paprika, salt, and pepper. Spread on a baking sheet and roast for 20 minutes, until tender. • Meanwhile, heat the remaining olive oil in a skillet over medium heat. Add the red bell pepper and red onion, sautéing until softened, about 5 minutes. • Add the black beans to the skillet and cook for another 3-5 minutes until heated through. • Warm the tortillas in a dry skillet or microwave. • To assemble, place half the roasted sweet potatoes, the black bean mixture, and fresh salsa onto each tortilla. Top with avocado slices and fresh cilantro. • Roll up the tortillas to form burritos. Serve immediately.
	NUTRITIONAL FACTS (per Serving): Calories: 380 | Total Fat: 17g | Saturated Fat: 2.5g | Fiber: 13g | Protein: 9g | Carbohydrate: 49g of which sugars: 7g | Calcium: 10% DV | Iron: 15% DV | Vitamin A: 320% DV

COCONUT YOGURT PARFAIT WITH GRANOLA

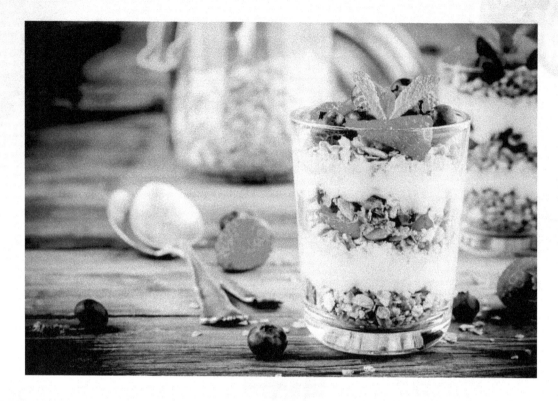

A creamy and delicious parfait made with coconut yogurt, layered with crunchy granola and fresh berries for a perfect start to your morning.

INGREDIENTS:	PREP TIME: 5 min	COOK TIME: 0 min	SERVINGS: 2 Servings
1 cup coconut yogurt 1/2 cup granola 1/2 cup fresh mixed berries (strawberries, blueberries, raspberries) 1 Tbsp chia seeds 1 Tbsp honey or maple syrup (optional)	**INSTRUCTIONS:** • In two glasses or bowls, layer 1/4 cup of coconut yogurt. • Add 2 Tbsp of granola and a layer of fresh berries. • Repeat the layers until all ingredients are used, finishing with a layer of berries on top. • Sprinkle chia seeds over the top and drizzle with honey or maple syrup if desired. • Serve immediately.		
	NUTRITIONAL FACTS (per Serving): Calories: 300 | Total Fat: 15g | Saturated Fat: 8g | Fiber: 7g | Protein: 5g | Carbohydrate: 38g of which sugars: 15g | Calcium: 10% DV | Iron: 10% DV | Vitamin C: 20% DV		

APPLE CINNAMON OVERNIGHT OATS

A delightful and convenient breakfast that's ready when you wake up, packed with the flavors of apple and cinnamon.

INGREDIENTS:	PREP TIME: 10 min	COOK TIME: 0 min	SERVINGS: 2 Servings

INGREDIENTS:	INSTRUCTIONS:
1 cup rolled oats 1 cup almond milk 1/2 cup unsweetened applesauce 1 apple, diced 1 Tbsp chia seeds 1 Tbsp maple syrup 1/2 tsp ground cinnamon 1/4 tsp vanilla extract 1/4 tsp nutmeg (optional) 2 Tbsp chopped walnuts (optional)	• In a bowl, combine rolled oats, almond milk, applesauce, chia seeds, maple syrup, cinnamon, vanilla extract, and nutmeg. • Mix well and divide the mixture into two jars or bowls. • Top with diced apple and chopped walnuts, if using. • Cover and refrigerate overnight. • Stir well before serving. Enjoy cold or warm it up in the microwave. **NUTRITIONAL FACTS (per Serving):** Calories: 300 | Total Fat: 8g | Saturated Fat: 1g | Fiber: 8g | Protein: 6g | Carbohydrate: 50g of which sugars: 15g | Calcium: 20% DV | Iron: 15% DV | Vitamin C: 10% DV

FRESH FRUIT SALAD WITH MINT

A refreshing and vibrant salad that combines a variety of fruits with a hint of mint, perfect for a light and nutritious breakfast.

INGREDIENTS:	PREP TIME: 15 min	COOK TIME: 0 min	SERVINGS: 2 Servings

INGREDIENTS:	INSTRUCTIONS:
1 cup strawberries, hulled and halved 1 cup blueberries 1 cup pineapple, diced 1 kiwi, peeled and sliced 1 orange, segmented 1 Tbsp fresh mint leaves, chopped 1 Tbsp lime juice 1 tsp honey (optional)	• In a large bowl, combine strawberries, blueberries, pineapple, kiwi, and orange segments. • Add the chopped mint leaves and gently toss to combine. • Drizzle with lime juice and honey, if using. • Mix well and serve immediately or refrigerate until ready to eat. **NUTRITIONAL FACTS (per Serving):** Calories: 140 | Total Fat: 0.5g | Saturated Fat: 0g | Fiber: 6g | Protein: 2g | Carbohydrate: 35g of which sugars: 25g | Vitamin C: 150% DV | Vitamin A: 10% DV | Calcium: 6% DV

TURMERIC AND GINGER SMOOTHIE

A vibrant and spicy smoothie packed with anti-inflammatory properties, perfect for a refreshing and health-boosting start to your day.

INGREDIENTS:	PREP TIME: 5 min	COOK TIME: 0 min	SERVINGS: 2 Servings

INGREDIENTS:	INSTRUCTIONS:
1 cup unsweetened almond milk 1 banana 1/2 cup frozen mango chunks 1/2 tsp ground turmeric 1/2 tsp fresh ginger, grated 1 Tbsp chia seeds 1 Tbsp honey or maple syrup 1/2 cup ice cubes	• In a blender, combine almond milk, banana, frozen mango, turmeric, ginger, chia seeds, honey or maple syrup, and ice cubes. • Blend on high until smooth and creamy. • Pour into two glasses and serve immediately. **NUTRITIONAL FACTS (per Serving):** Calories: 190 | Total Fat: 5g | Saturated Fat: 0.5g | Fiber: 5g | Protein: 3g | Carbohydrate: 37g of which sugars: 22g | Vitamin C: 40% DV | Calcium: 20% DV | Iron: 6% DV

WARM BUCKWHEAT PORRIDGE WITH BERRIES

A hearty and warming porridge made with buckwheat, providing a nutritious start to your day, topped with fresh berries for extra flavor.

INGREDIENTS:	PREP TIME: 5 min	COOK TIME: 15 min	SERVINGS: 2 Servings

INGREDIENTS:	INSTRUCTIONS:
1/2 cup buckwheat groats 1 1/2 cups water 1/2 cup almond milk 1 Tbsp chia seeds 1 Tbsp maple syrup 1/2 tsp ground cinnamon 1/2 cup mixed berries (blueberries, raspberries, strawberries) 1 Tbsp chopped nuts (optional)	• Rinse buckwheat groats under cold water. • In a medium saucepan, combine buckwheat groats and water. Bring to a boil, then reduce heat and simmer for 10 minutes, or until tender. • Stir in almond milk, chia seeds, maple syrup, and cinnamon. Cook for an additional 5 minutes, stirring frequently, until the porridge thickens. • Divide the porridge into two bowls and top with mixed berries and chopped nuts, if using. Serve warm. **NUTRITIONAL FACTS (per Serving):** Calories: 260 | Total Fat: 6g | Saturated Fat: 0.5g | Fiber: 8g | Protein: 7g | Carbohydrate: 48g of which sugars: 10g | Calcium: 15% DV | Iron: 15% DV | Vitamin C: 10% DV

VEGAN BANANA NUT MUFFINS

Delicious and moist muffins made with ripe bananas and crunchy nuts, perfect for a healthy and satisfying breakfast.

INGREDIENTS:	PREP TIME: 10 min	COOK TIME: 20 min	SERVINGS: 2 Servings
1 cup whole wheat flour 1 tsp baking powder 1/2 tsp baking soda 1/4 tsp salt 2 ripe bananas, mashed 1/4 cup maple syrup 1/4 cup unsweetened applesauce 1 tsp vanilla extract 1/4 cup chopped walnuts or pecans	**INSTRUCTIONS:** • Preheat oven to 350°F (175°C) and line a muffin tin with paper liners. • In a large bowl, whisk together whole wheat flour, baking powder, baking soda, and salt. • In a separate bowl, mix mashed bananas, maple syrup, applesauce, and vanilla extract until well combined. • Add the wet ingredients to the dry ingredients and mix until just combined. Fold in chopped nuts. • Divide the batter evenly among the muffin cups. • Bake for 18-20 minutes, or until a toothpick inserted into the center comes out clean. Allow to cool slightly before serving.		
	NUTRITIONAL FACTS (per Serving): Calories: 210 | Total Fat: 6g | Saturated Fat: 0.5g | Fiber: 5g | Protein: 4g | Carbohydrate: 38g of which sugars: 12g | Vitamin C: 6% DV | Calcium: 10% DV | Iron: 8% DV		

KALE AND SWEET POTATO HASH

A hearty and nutritious hash made with kale and sweet potatoes, perfect for a savory breakfast that's both satisfying and healthful.

INGREDIENTS:	PREP TIME: 10 min	COOK TIME: 20 min	SERVINGS: 2 Servings
1 medium sweet potato, peeled and diced 1 Tbsp olive oil 1 small red onion, diced 1 red bell pepper, diced 2 cups kale, chopped 1/2 tsp smoked paprika 1/2 tsp ground cumin Salt and pepper to taste 1 avocado, sliced (for serving)	**INSTRUCTIONS:** • Heat olive oil in a large skillet over medium heat. • Add diced sweet potato and cook for 10 minutes, stirring occasionally. • Add red onion and red bell pepper, cooking for another 5 minutes until softened. • Stir in kale, smoked paprika, cumin, salt, and pepper. Cook until kale is wilted, about 3 minutes. • Serve hot, topped with avocado slices.		
	NUTRITIONAL FACTS (per Serving): Calories: 250 | Total Fat: 12g | Saturated Fat: 1.5g | Fiber: 8g | Protein: 4g | Carbohydrate: 34g of which sugars: 8g | Vitamin A: 370% DV | Vitamin C: 120% DV | Calcium: 15% DV | Iron: 10% DV		

STEEL-CUT OATS WITH MIXED NUTS AND HONEY

A hearty and nutritious breakfast bowl featuring steel-cut oats, topped with a mix of nuts and a drizzle of honey for a touch of sweetness.

INGREDIENTS:	PREP TIME: 5 min	COOK TIME: 25 min	SERVINGS: 2 Servings

INGREDIENTS:	INSTRUCTIONS:
1/2 cup steel-cut oats 2 cups water 1/4 tsp salt 1/4 cup mixed nuts (almonds, walnuts, pecans), chopped 1 Tbsp honey 1/2 tsp ground cinnamon 1/4 cup almond milk (optional, for serving)	• In a medium saucepan, bring water to a boil and add salt. • Stir in the steel-cut oats, reduce heat to low, and simmer for 20-25 minutes, stirring occasionally, until the oats are tender. • Divide the cooked oats into two bowls. • Top with mixed nuts, a drizzle of honey, and ground cinnamon. • Add a splash of almond milk if desired. Serve warm.

NUTRITIONAL FACTS (per Serving): Calories: 250 | Total Fat: 10g | Saturated Fat: 1g | Fiber: 6g | Protein: 6g | Carbohydrate: 36g of which sugars: 10g | Iron: 10% DV | Calcium: 8% DV | Vitamin E: 10% DV

CARROT CAKE BREAKFAST BARS

Delicious and moist breakfast bars that capture the flavors of carrot cake, perfect for a grab-and-go morning meal.

INGREDIENTS:	PREP TIME: 10 min	COOK TIME: 30 min	SERVINGS: 2 Servings

INGREDIENTS:	INSTRUCTIONS:
1 cup rolled oats 1/2 cup whole wheat flour 1 tsp baking powder 1/2 tsp ground cinnamon 1/4 tsp ground nutmeg 1/4 tsp salt 1 cup grated carrots 1/4 cup maple syrup 1/4 cup unsweetened applesauce 1/4 cup almond milk 1 tsp vanilla extract 1/4 cup chopped walnuts or pecans	• Preheat oven to 350°F (175°C) and line a baking dish with parchment paper. • In a large bowl, mix rolled oats, whole wheat flour, baking powder, cinnamon, nutmeg, and salt. • In another bowl, combine grated carrots, maple syrup, applesauce, almond milk, and vanilla extract. • Add the wet ingredients to the dry ingredients and mix until well combined. Fold in chopped nuts. • Pour the batter into the prepared baking dish and spread evenly. • Bake for 25-30 minutes, or until a toothpick inserted into the center comes out clean. Allow to cool before cutting into bars.

NUTRITIONAL FACTS (per Serving): Calories: 280 | Total Fat: 9g | Saturated Fat: 1g | Fiber: 5g | Protein: 5g | Carbohydrate: 44g of which sugars: 12g | Vitamin A: 80% DV | Iron: 10% DV | Calcium: 10% DV

LEMON AND CHIA SEED SCONES

Light and zesty scones with the added crunch of chia seeds, perfect for a refreshing breakfast treat.

INGREDIENTS:	PREP TIME: 10 min	COOK TIME: 20 min	SERVINGS: 2 Servings

INGREDIENTS:	INSTRUCTIONS:
1 cup whole wheat flour	• Preheat oven to 375°F (190°C) and line a baking sheet with parchment paper.
1/2 cup almond flour	• In a large bowl, mix whole wheat flour, almond flour, chia seeds, coconut sugar, baking powder, baking soda, and salt.
2 Tbsp chia seeds	
2 Tbsp coconut sugar	• Cut in the solid coconut oil until the mixture resembles coarse crumbs.
1 tsp baking powder	• In a separate bowl, mix almond milk, lemon zest, lemon juice, and vanilla extract.
1/4 tsp baking soda	
1/4 tsp salt	• Add the wet ingredients to the dry ingredients and stir until just combined.
1/4 cup coconut oil, solid	• Turn the dough out onto a lightly floured surface and shape it into a circle about 1 inch thick. Cut into 6 wedges and place on the prepared baking sheet.
1/2 cup almond milk	
Zest of 1 lemon	
1 Tbsp lemon juice	• Bake for 18-20 minutes, or until golden brown. Allow to cool slightly before serving.
1/2 tsp vanilla extract	

NUTRITIONAL FACTS (per Serving): Calories: 270 | Total Fat: 16g | Saturated Fat: 6g | Fiber: 5g | Protein: 6g | Carbohydrate: 28g of which sugars: 6g | Vitamin C: 6% DV | Calcium: 8% DV | Iron: 10% DV

SPINACH AND MUSHROOM BREAKFAST WRAP

A savory and nutritious breakfast wrap filled with sautéed spinach and mushrooms, perfect for a quick and satisfying morning meal.

INGREDIENTS:	PREP TIME: 10 min	COOK TIME: 10 min	SERVINGS: 2 Servings

INGREDIENTS:	INSTRUCTIONS:
1 Tbsp olive oil	• Heat olive oil in a skillet over medium heat.
1 small red onion, diced	• Add diced red onion and sliced mushrooms, cooking until softened, about 5 minutes.
1 cup mushrooms, sliced	
2 cups spinach leaves, chopped	• Stir in chopped spinach, garlic powder, smoked paprika, salt, and pepper. Cook until spinach is wilted, about 2 minutes.
1/2 tsp garlic powder	• Warm the tortillas in a dry skillet or microwave.
1/2 tsp smoked paprika	• Spread 2 Tbsp of hummus on each tortilla.
Salt and pepper to taste	
2 large whole wheat tortillas	• Divide the spinach and mushroom mixture between the two tortillas and top with avocado slices.
1/4 cup hummus	• Roll up the tortillas to form wraps. Serve immediately.
1 avocado, sliced	

NUTRITIONAL FACTS (per Serving): Calories: 310 | Total Fat: 18g | Saturated Fat: 3g | Fiber: 9g | Protein: 7g | Carbohydrate: 35g of which sugars: 4g | Vitamin A: 80% DV | Vitamin C: 30% DV | Calcium: 10% DV | Iron: 15% DV

2. MID-MORNING SNACKS

COCONUT AND DATE BLISS BALLS

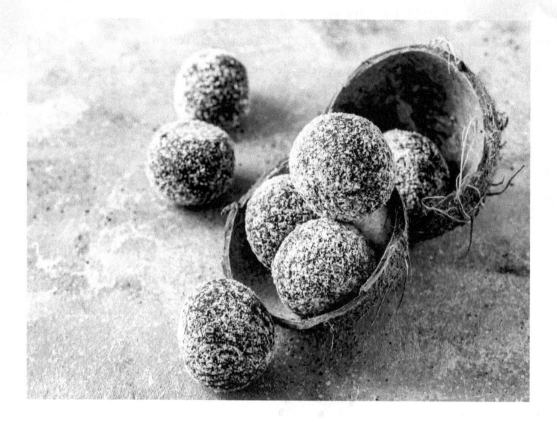

Delicious and energy-boosting bliss balls made with coconut and dates, perfect for a quick and healthy snack.

INGREDIENTS:	PREP TIME: 10 min	COOK TIME: 0 min	SERVINGS: 2 Servings

INGREDIENTS:	INSTRUCTIONS:
1/2 cup pitted dates	
1/4 cup almonds	• In a food processor, combine pitted dates, almonds, shredded coconut, chia seeds, cocoa powder (if using), vanilla extract, and coconut oil.
1/4 cup shredded coconut	
1 Tbsp chia seeds	• Process until the mixture is well combined and sticky.
1 Tbsp cocoa powder (optional)	• Roll the mixture into small balls (about 1 inch in diameter).
1 tsp vanilla extract	• Place the bliss balls in the refrigerator for at least 30 minutes to set before serving.
1 Tbsp coconut oil	

NUTRITIONAL FACTS (per Serving): Calories: 200 | Total Fat: 12g | Saturated Fat: 6g | Fiber: 5g | Protein: 3g | Carbohydrate: 24g of which sugars: 18g | Calcium: 4% DV | Iron: 6% DV | Vitamin E: 4% DV

APPLE SLICES WITH ALMOND BUTTER

A simple and satisfying snack combining the crispness of apples with the creamy richness of almond butter.

INGREDIENTS:	PREP TIME: 5 min	COOK TIME: 0 min	SERVINGS: 2 Servings
2 apples, sliced 4 Tbsp almond butter 1 tsp chia seeds (optional) 1/2 tsp ground cinnamon (optional)	**INSTRUCTIONS:** • Core and slice the apples. • Arrange the apple slices on a plate. • Spread 2 Tbsp of almond butter on each serving of apple slices. • Sprinkle with chia seeds and ground cinnamon if desired. • Serve immediately.		
	NUTRITIONAL FACTS (per Serving): Calories: 220 | Total Fat: 14g | Saturated Fat: 1g | Fiber: 6g | Protein: 4g | Carbohydrate: 24g of which sugars: 16g | Vitamin C: 10% DV | Calcium: 6% DV | Iron: 4% DV		

MIXED BERRY AND NUT ENERGY BARS

Nutritious and delicious energy bars packed with berries and nuts, perfect for a quick mid-morning snack.

INGREDIENTS:	PREP TIME: 10 min	COOK TIME: 20 min	SERVINGS: 2 Servings
1/2 cup rolled oats 1/4 cup almonds, chopped 1/4 cup walnuts, chopped 1/4 cup dried mixed berries (blueberries, cranberries, raisins) 2 Tbsp chia seeds 2 Tbsp honey or maple syrup 1/4 cup almond butter 1/2 tsp vanilla extract	**INSTRUCTIONS:** • Preheat oven to 350°F (175°C) and line a baking dish with parchment paper. • In a bowl, mix rolled oats, almonds, walnuts, dried berries, and chia seeds. • In a saucepan, warm the honey or maple syrup and almond butter over low heat until smooth. Stir in vanilla extract. • Pour the almond butter mixture over the dry ingredients and mix until well combined. • Press the mixture firmly into the prepared baking dish. • Bake for 20 minutes or until golden brown. Allow to cool before cutting into bars.		
	NUTRITIONAL FACTS (per Serving): Calories: 280 | Total Fat: 16g | Saturated Fat: 2g | Fiber: 6g | Protein: 6g | Carbohydrate: 28g of which sugars: 12g | Calcium: 8% DV | Iron: 8% DV | Vitamin E: 10% DV		

HUMMUS WITH CARROT AND CUCUMBER STICKS

A refreshing and nutritious snack that pairs creamy hummus with crisp vegetable sticks.

INGREDIENTS:	PREP TIME: 10 min	COOK TIME: 0 min	SERVINGS: 2 Servings

INGREDIENTS:	INSTRUCTIONS:
1 cup hummus 2 large carrots, peeled and cut into sticks 1 cucumber, sliced into sticks	• Arrange the carrot and cucumber sticks on a plate. • Serve with a bowl of hummus on the side. • Dip the vegetable sticks into the hummus and enjoy.

NUTRITIONAL FACTS (per Serving): Calories: 180 | Total Fat: 9g | Saturated Fat: 1g | Fiber: 6g | Protein: 5g | Carbohydrate: 20g of which sugars: 6g | Vitamin A: 210% DV | Vitamin C: 15% DV | Calcium: 6% DV | Iron: 8% DV

FRESH PINEAPPLE AND MINT SALAD

A refreshing and tropical mid-morning snack combining the sweetness of pineapple with the coolness of mint.

INGREDIENTS:	PREP TIME: 10 min	COOK TIME: 0 min	SERVINGS: 2 Servings

INGREDIENTS:	INSTRUCTIONS:
2 cups fresh pineapple, diced 1 Tbsp fresh mint leaves, chopped 1 Tbsp lime juice 1 tsp honey (optional)	• In a large bowl, combine diced pineapple and chopped mint leaves. • Drizzle with lime juice and honey if desired. • Toss gently to mix well. • Serve immediately or refrigerate until ready to eat.

NUTRITIONAL FACTS (per Serving): Calories: 80 | Total Fat: 0.5g | Saturated Fat: 0g | Fiber: 2g | Protein: 1g | Carbohydrate: 21g of which sugars: 16g | Vitamin C: 100% DV | Calcium: 2% DV | Iron: 2% DV

EDAMAME WITH SEA SALT

A simple, protein-packed snack that's both tasty and nutritious, perfect for mid-morning cravings.

INGREDIENTS:	PREP TIME: 5 min	COOK TIME: 5 min	SERVINGS: 2 Servings
2 cups edamame in pods 1 tsp sea salt 1 lemon wedge (optional)	**INSTRUCTIONS:** • Bring a pot of water to a boil and add the edamame. Cook for 5 minutes. • Drain the edamame and transfer to a bowl. • Sprinkle with sea salt and toss to coat. • Squeeze a lemon wedge over the edamame if desired. Serve warm.		
	NUTRITIONAL FACTS (per Serving): Calories: 120 | Total Fat: 5g | Saturated Fat: 0.5g | Fiber: 6g | Protein: 10g | Carbohydrate: 10g of which sugars: 2g | Calcium: 4% DV | Iron: 10% DV | Vitamin C: 8% DV		

SPICED PUMPKIN SEEDS

A crunchy and flavorful snack, these spiced pumpkin seeds are perfect for a nutritious mid-morning bite.

INGREDIENTS:	PREP TIME: 5 min	COOK TIME: 15 min	SERVINGS: 2 Servings
1 cup pumpkin seeds 1 Tbsp olive oil 1/2 tsp smoked paprika 1/2 tsp ground cumin 1/4 tsp cayenne pepper (optional) 1/2 tsp sea salt	**INSTRUCTIONS:** • Preheat oven to 300°F (150°C) and line a baking sheet with parchment paper. • In a bowl, mix pumpkin seeds with olive oil, smoked paprika, ground cumin, cayenne pepper (if using), and sea salt. • Spread the seeds evenly on the prepared baking sheet. • Bake for 15 minutes, stirring halfway through, until golden and crispy. • Allow to cool before serving.		
	NUTRITIONAL FACTS (per Serving): Calories: 180 | Total Fat: 14g | Saturated Fat: 2g | Fiber: 3g | Protein: 8g | Carbohydrate: 6g of which sugars: 1g | Calcium: 2% DV | Iron: 15% DV | Vitamin E: 4% DV		

GREEK YOGURT WITH HONEY AND WALNUTS

A creamy and satisfying snack that combines the richness of Greek yogurt with the sweetness of honey and the crunch of walnuts.

INGREDIENTS:	PREP TIME: 5 min	COOK TIME: 0 min	SERVINGS: 2 Servings
1 cup Greek yogurt 2 Tbsp honey 1/4 cup walnuts, chopped 1/2 tsp ground cinnamon (optional)	**INSTRUCTIONS:** • Divide the Greek yogurt into two bowls. • Drizzle 1 Tbsp of honey over each serving of yogurt. • Sprinkle each with 2 Tbsp of chopped walnuts. • Add a pinch of ground cinnamon if desired. • Serve immediately.		

NUTRITIONAL FACTS (per Serving): Calories: 220 | Total Fat: 10g | Saturated Fat: 2g | Fiber: 2g | Protein: 15g | Carbohydrate: 22g of which sugars: 17g | Calcium: 15% DV | Iron: 4% DV | Vitamin C: 0% DV

BAKED ZUCCHINI CHIPS

A healthy and crunchy snack, these baked zucchini chips are a perfect alternative to traditional chips.

INGREDIENTS:	PREP TIME: 10 min	COOK TIME: 20 min	SERVINGS: 2 Servings
2 medium zucchinis, thinly sliced 1 Tbsp olive oil 1/2 tsp sea salt 1/2 tsp garlic powder 1/4 tsp smoked paprika	**INSTRUCTIONS:** • Preheat oven to 425°F (220°C) and line a baking sheet with parchment paper. • In a bowl, toss zucchini slices with olive oil, sea salt, garlic powder, and smoked paprika. • Arrange the zucchini slices in a single layer on the prepared baking sheet. • Bake for 15-20 minutes, or until crispy and golden brown, turning halfway through. • Allow to cool slightly before serving.		

NUTRITIONAL FACTS (per Serving): Calories: 90 | Total Fat: 5g | Saturated Fat: 0.5g | Fiber: 2g | Protein: 2g | Carbohydrate: 10g of which sugars: 3g | Calcium: 2% DV | Iron: 4% DV | Vitamin A: 6% DV | Vitamin C: 20% DV

3. LUNCH

ZUCCHINI NOODLES WITH PESTO AND CHERRY TOMATOES

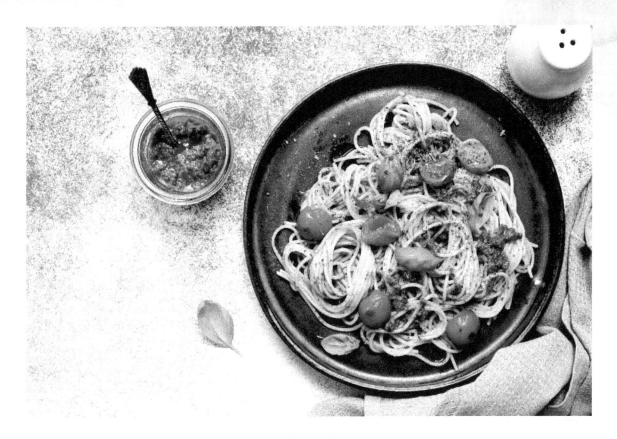

A light and flavorful dish featuring zucchini noodles tossed with fresh pesto and juicy cherry tomatoes.

INGREDIENTS:	PREP TIME: 15 min	COOK TIME: 5 min	SERVINGS: 2 Servings
2 medium zucchinis, spiralized 1 cup cherry tomatoes, halved 1/4 cup fresh basil leaves 2 Tbsp pine nuts 1 clove garlic 2 Tbsp olive oil 1 Tbsp lemon juice Salt and pepper to taste 1/4 cup grated Parmesan cheese (optional)	**INSTRUCTIONS:** • In a food processor, blend basil leaves, pine nuts, garlic, olive oil, lemon juice, salt, and pepper until smooth to make the pesto. • In a large pan, lightly sauté the zucchini noodles over medium heat for 2–3 minutes until just tender. • Remove from heat and toss with cherry tomatoes and pesto. • Serve immediately, topped with grated Parmesan cheese if desired. **NUTRITIONAL FACTS (per Serving):** Calories: 220 | Total Fat: 18g | Saturated Fat: 2.5g | Fiber: 4g | Protein: 6g | Carbohydrate: 12g of which sugars: 6g | Vitamin A: 15% DV | Vitamin C: 40% DV | Calcium: 8% DV | Iron: 10% DV		

QUINOA AND CHICKPEA SALAD WITH LEMON TAHINI DRESSING

A light and refreshing salad packed with protein and flavor, perfect for a nutritious lunch.

INGREDIENTS:	PREP TIME: 15 min	COOK TIME: 15 min	SERVINGS: 2 Servings

INGREDIENTS:	INSTRUCTIONS:
1/2 cup quinoa, rinsed 1 cup water 1 cup chickpeas, cooked and drained 1/2 cucumber, diced 1/2 red bell pepper, diced 1/4 red onion, finely chopped 1/4 cup fresh parsley, chopped	• In a medium saucepan, combine quinoa and water. Bring to a boil, then reduce heat and simmer for 15 minutes or until the quinoa is cooked and water is absorbed. Let cool. • In a large bowl, combine cooked quinoa, chickpeas, cucumber, red bell pepper, red onion, and parsley. • In a small bowl, whisk together tahini, lemon juice, olive oil, water, garlic, salt, and pepper until smooth. • Pour the dressing over the salad and toss to coat. • Serve immediately or refrigerate until ready to eat.
	NUTRITIONAL FACTS (per Serving): Calories: 320 | Total Fat: 14g | Saturated Fat: 2g | Fiber: 9g | Protein: 11g | Carbohydrate: 40g of which sugars: 4g | Vitamin A: 20% DV | Vitamin C: 60% DV | Calcium: 10% DV | Iron: 20% DV

LENTIL AND VEGETABLE SOUP

A hearty and comforting soup filled with lentils and vegetables, perfect for a wholesome lunch.

INGREDIENTS:	PREP TIME: 10 min	COOK TIME: 30 min	SERVINGS: 2 Servings

INGREDIENTS:	INSTRUCTIONS:
1 cup lentils, rinsed 1 Tbsp olive oil 1 small onion, diced 2 carrots, diced 2 celery stalks, diced 1 red bell pepper, diced 2 cloves garlic, minced 4 cups vegetable broth 1 tsp ground cumin 1/2 tsp smoked paprika Salt and pepper to taste 2 cups spinach leaves, chopped	• In a large pot, heat olive oil over medium heat. Add onion, carrots, celery, and red bell pepper. Sauté until vegetables are softened, about 5 minutes. • Add garlic and cook for 1 minute until fragrant. • Stir in lentils, vegetable broth, cumin, smoked paprika, salt, and pepper. Bring to a boil. • Reduce heat and simmer for 20-25 minutes, or until lentils are tender. • Stir in chopped spinach and cook for an additional 2-3 minutes until wilted. • Serve hot.
	NUTRITIONAL FACTS (per Serving): Calories: 250 | Total Fat: 7g | Saturated Fat: 1g | Fiber: 12g | Protein: 12g | Carbohydrate: 36g of which sugars: 6g | Vitamin A: 100% DV | Vitamin C: 50% DV | Calcium: 10% DV | Iron: 25% DV

SWEET POTATO AND BLACK BEAN TACOS

These delicious and nutritious tacos are filled with roasted sweet potatoes and black beans, topped with a tangy avocado sauce.

INGREDIENTS:	PREP TIME: 15 min	COOK TIME: 25 min	SERVINGS: 2 Servings

INGREDIENTS:

1 medium sweet potato, peeled and diced

1 Tbsp olive oil

1/2 tsp smoked paprika

1/2 tsp ground cumin

Salt and pepper to taste

1 cup black beans, cooked and drained

4 small whole wheat tortillas

1/2 cup shredded red cabbage

1/4 cup chopped fresh cilantro

1 ripe avocado

1/4 cup plain Greek yogurt (or a dairy-free alternative)

1 Tbsp lime juice

1 clove garlic, minced

Salt and pepper to taste

INSTRUCTIONS:

- Preheat oven to 400°F (200°C). Toss diced sweet potatoes with olive oil, smoked paprika, ground cumin, salt, and pepper. Spread on a baking sheet and roast for 25 minutes, or until tender.

- In a bowl, mash the avocado and mix with Greek yogurt, lime juice, minced garlic, salt, and pepper until smooth.

- Warm the tortillas in a dry skillet or microwave.

- Fill each tortilla with roasted sweet potatoes, black beans, shredded red cabbage, and chopped cilantro.

- Drizzle with avocado sauce and serve immediately.

NUTRITIONAL FACTS (per Serving): Calories: 350 | Total Fat: 16g | Saturated Fat: 2.5g | Fiber: 12g | Protein: 9g | Carbohydrate: 46g of which sugars: 6g | Vitamin A: 200% DV | Vitamin C: 35% DV | Calcium: 10% DV | Iron: 15% DV

SPINACH AND AVOCADO SALAD WITH POMEGRANATE SEEDS

A vibrant and nutritious salad combining the creaminess of avocado with the freshness of spinach and the burst of pomegranate seeds.

INGREDIENTS:	PREP TIME: 10 min	COOK TIME: 0 min	SERVINGS: 2 Servings

INGREDIENTS:

4 cups fresh spinach leaves

1 avocado, sliced

1/2 cup pomegranate seeds

1/4 red onion, thinly sliced

1/4 cup walnuts, chopped

2 Tbsp olive oil

1 Tbsp balsamic vinegar

Salt and pepper to taste

INSTRUCTIONS:

- In a large bowl, combine spinach leaves, avocado slices, pomegranate seeds, red onion, and walnuts.

- In a small bowl, whisk together olive oil, balsamic vinegar, salt, and pepper.

- Drizzle the dressing over the salad and toss gently to combine.

- Serve immediately.

NUTRITIONAL FACTS (per Serving): Calories: 280 | Total Fat: 22g | Saturated Fat: 3g | Fiber: 8g | Protein: 4g | Carbohydrate: 20g of which sugars: 10g | Vitamin A: 80% DV | Vitamin C: 30% DV | Calcium: 10% DV | Iron: 15% DV

BAKED FALAFEL WITH TZATZIKI SAUCE

Enjoy these delicious and healthy baked falafels, paired with a refreshing tzatziki sauce.

INGREDIENTS:	PREP TIME: 20 min	COOK TIME: 25 min	SERVINGS: 2 Servings

INGREDIENTS:

1 cup chickpeas, cooked and drained

1/4 cup red onion, finely chopped

2 cloves garlic, minced

1/4 cup fresh parsley, chopped

1 tsp ground cumin

1 tsp ground coriander

1/2 tsp baking powder

2 Tbsp whole wheat flour

Salt and pepper to taste

2 Tbsp olive oil (for brushing)

1/2 cup Greek yogurt

1/2 cucumber, grated and drained

1 clove garlic, minced

1 Tbsp lemon juice

1 Tbsp fresh dill, chopped

Salt and pepper to taste

INSTRUCTIONS:

- Preheat oven to 375°F (190°C) and line a baking sheet with parchment paper.

- In a food processor, combine chickpeas, red onion, garlic, parsley, cumin, coriander, baking powder, flour, salt, and pepper. Pulse until well combined but still slightly chunky.

- Form the mixture into small patties and place on the prepared baking sheet.

- Brush the patties with olive oil and bake for 25 minutes, flipping halfway through.

- Meanwhile, mix all tzatziki sauce ingredients in a bowl.

- Serve the falafel with tzatziki sauce on the side.

NUTRITIONAL FACTS (per Serving): Calories: 280 | Total Fat: 12g | Saturated Fat: 2g | Fiber: 9g | Protein: 11g | Carbohydrate: 32g of which sugars: 4g | Vitamin A: 8% DV | Vitamin C: 20% DV | Calcium: 10% DV | Iron: 15% DV

CAULIFLOWER RICE STIR-FRY WITH TOFU

A flavorful and nutritious stir-fry made with cauliflower rice and tofu, perfect for a light and healthy lunch.

INGREDIENTS:	PREP TIME: 15 min	COOK TIME: 15 min	SERVINGS: 2 Servings

INGREDIENTS:

1 block (14 oz) firm tofu, drained and cubed

1 Tbsp olive oil

2 cups cauliflower rice

1 red bell pepper, diced

1 cup broccoli florets

1 small carrot, julienned

2 cloves garlic, minced

1 Tbsp soy sauce (or tamari for gluten-free)

1 tsp sesame oil

1/2 tsp ground ginger

1/4 cup fresh cilantro, chopped

INSTRUCTIONS:

- Heat olive oil in a large skillet over medium heat. Add tofu cubes and cook until golden brown on all sides, about 5-7 minutes. Remove tofu from the skillet and set aside.

- In the same skillet, add cauliflower rice, red bell pepper, broccoli, carrot, and garlic. Cook for 5-7 minutes until vegetables are tender.

- Stir in soy sauce, sesame oil, and ground ginger. Add the tofu back to the skillet and toss to combine.

- Cook for an additional 2 minutes until everything is well heated.

- Garnish with fresh cilantro and serve immediately.

NUTRITIONAL FACTS (per Serving): Calories: 300 | Total Fat: 18g | Saturated Fat: 3g | Fiber: 7g | Protein: 18g | Carbohydrate: 18g of which sugars: 6g | Vitamin A: 70% DV | Vitamin C: 90% DV | Calcium: 20% DV | Iron: 20% DV

MEDITERRANEAN STUFFED BELL PEPPERS

Colorful bell peppers stuffed with a savory mix of quinoa, chickpeas, and Mediterranean flavors, perfect for a healthy and filling lunch.

INGREDIENTS:	PREP TIME: 15 min	COOK TIME: 30 min	SERVINGS: 2 Servings

INGREDIENTS	INSTRUCTIONS
2 large bell peppers, halved and seeded 1/2 cup quinoa, cooked 1/2 cup chickpeas, cooked and drained 1/4 cup Kalamata olives, chopped 1/4 cup cherry tomatoes, diced 2 Tbsp red onion, finely chopped 2 Tbsp fresh parsley, chopped 2 Tbsp feta cheese, crumbled (optional) 1 Tbsp olive oil 1 Tbsp lemon juice Salt and pepper to taste	**INSTRUCTIONS:** • Preheat oven to 375°F (190°C). • In a large bowl, combine cooked quinoa, chickpeas, olives, cherry tomatoes, red onion, parsley, feta cheese (if using), olive oil, lemon juice, salt, and pepper. • Stuff each bell pepper half with the quinoa mixture. • Place the stuffed peppers in a baking dish and cover with foil. • Bake for 25-30 minutes, or until the peppers are tender. • Serve warm. **NUTRITIONAL FACTS (per Serving):** Calories: 260 | Total Fat: 10g | Saturated Fat: 2g | Fiber: 8g | Protein: 8g | Carbohydrate: 35g of which sugars: 8g | Vitamin A: 100% DV | Vitamin C: 200% DV | Calcium: 10% DV | Iron: 15% DV

VEGAN BUDDHA BOWL WITH TAHINI DRESSING

A colorful and nutritious Buddha bowl filled with a variety of plant-based ingredients and drizzled with a creamy tahini dressing.

INGREDIENTS:	PREP TIME: 15 min	COOK TIME: 20 min	SERVINGS: 2 Servings

INGREDIENTS	INSTRUCTIONS
1/2 cup quinoa, cooked 1 cup chickpeas, cooked and drained 1 cup roasted sweet potatoes, diced 1/2 cup red cabbage, shredded 1/2 cup carrots, shredded 1 avocado, sliced 1/4 cup fresh cilantro, chopped 2 Tbsp tahini 1 Tbsp lemon juice 1 Tbsp maple syrup 2 Tbsp water 1 clove garlic, minced Salt and pepper to taste	**INSTRUCTIONS:** • In a large bowl, arrange the quinoa, chickpeas, roasted sweet potatoes, red cabbage, carrots, avocado, and cilantro. • In a small bowl, whisk together tahini, lemon juice, maple syrup, water, garlic, salt, and pepper until smooth. • Drizzle the tahini dressing over the Buddha bowl. • Serve immediately. **NUTRITIONAL FACTS (per Serving):** Calories: 350 | Total Fat: 18g | Saturated Fat: 2.5g | Fiber: 12g | Protein: 10g | Carbohydrate: 40g of which sugars: 8g | Vitamin A: 150% DV | Vitamin C: 60% DV | Calcium: 10% DV | Iron: 15% DV

ROASTED VEGETABLE AND HUMMUS WRAP

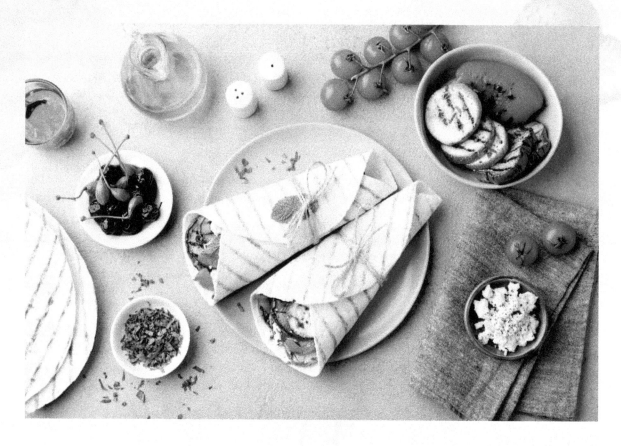

A wholesome and flavorful wrap filled with roasted vegetables and creamy hummus, perfect for a healthy and satisfying lunch.

INGREDIENTS:	PREP TIME: 10 min	COOK TIME: 25 min	SERVINGS: 2 Servings

INGREDIENTS:	
1 small zucchini, sliced	**INSTRUCTIONS:**
1 red bell pepper, sliced	
1 small eggplant, sliced	• Preheat oven to 425°F (220°C). Toss zucchini, red bell pepper, and eggplant slices with olive oil, salt, pepper, dried oregano, and garlic powder. Spread on a baking sheet and roast for 20-25 minutes, or until tender.
1 Tbsp olive oil	
Salt and pepper to taste	• Warm the tortillas in a dry skillet or microwave.
1/2 tsp dried oregano	
1/2 tsp garlic powder	• Spread 1/4 cup of hummus on each tortilla.
2 large whole wheat tortillas	• Top with roasted vegetables, fresh spinach leaves, and crumbled feta cheese if using.
1/2 cup hummus	• Roll up the tortillas to form wraps. Serve immediately.
1 cup fresh spinach leaves	
1/4 cup crumbled feta cheese (optional)	**NUTRITIONAL FACTS (per Serving):** Calories: 320 | Total Fat: 14g | Saturated Fat: 2g | Fiber: 9g | Protein: 9g | Carbohydrate: 40g of which sugars: 7g | Vitamin A: 30% DV | Vitamin C: 90% DV | Calcium: 10% DV | Iron: 15% DV

WILD RICE AND MUSHROOM PILAF

A hearty and flavorful pilaf made with wild rice and mushrooms, perfect for a satisfying lunch.

INGREDIENTS:	PREP TIME: 10 min	COOK TIME: 35 min	SERVINGS: 2 Servings

INGREDIENTS	INSTRUCTIONS
1/2 cup wild rice 1 cup vegetable broth 1 Tbsp olive oil 1 small onion, diced 2 cloves garlic, minced 1 cup mushrooms, sliced 1/2 cup celery, diced 1/4 cup dried cranberries 1/4 cup chopped walnuts Salt and pepper to taste 2 Tbsp fresh parsley, chopped	**INSTRUCTIONS:** • Rinse the wild rice under cold water. In a medium saucepan, combine wild rice and vegetable broth. Bring to a boil, then reduce heat and simmer for 30-35 minutes, or until the rice is tender. • In a large skillet, heat olive oil over medium heat. Add onion and garlic, and sauté until fragrant, about 3 minutes. • Add mushrooms and celery, and cook for another 5 minutes until softened. • Stir in cooked wild rice, dried cranberries, chopped walnuts, salt, and pepper. Cook for 2-3 minutes until heated through. • Garnish with fresh parsley and serve warm. **NUTRITIONAL FACTS (per Serving):** Calories: 320 | Total Fat: 14g | Saturated Fat: 1.5g | Fiber: 6g | Protein: 8g | Carbohydrate: 44g of which sugars: 8g | Vitamin A: 8% DV | Vitamin C: 10% DV | Calcium: 6% DV | Iron: 15% DV

CHICKPEA AND KALE STEW

A hearty and nutritious stew made with chickpeas and kale, packed with flavor and perfect for a comforting lunch.

INGREDIENTS:	PREP TIME: 10 min	COOK TIME: 25 min	SERVINGS: 2 Servings

INGREDIENTS	INSTRUCTIONS
1 Tbsp olive oil 1 small onion, diced 2 cloves garlic, minced 1 carrot, diced 1 celery stalk, diced 1 cup chickpeas, cooked and drained 4 cups kale, chopped 2 cups vegetable broth 1 can (14.5 oz) diced tomatoes 1 tsp ground cumin 1/2 tsp smoked paprika Salt and pepper to taste	**INSTRUCTIONS:** • Heat olive oil in a large pot over medium heat. Add onion and garlic, and sauté until fragrant, about 3 minutes. • Add carrot and celery, and cook for another 5 minutes until vegetables are softened. • Stir in chickpeas, kale, vegetable broth, diced tomatoes, cumin, smoked paprika, salt, and pepper. • Bring to a boil, then reduce heat and simmer for 15-20 minutes until the flavors are well combined and the kale is tender. • Serve hot. **NUTRITIONAL FACTS (per Serving):** Calories: 220 | Total Fat: 7g | Saturated Fat: 1g | Fiber: 10g | Protein: 8g | Carbohydrate: 30g of which sugars: 8g | Vitamin A: 200% DV | Vitamin C: 100% DV | Calcium: 15% DV | Iron: 20% DV

GRILLED PORTOBELLO MUSHROOM SANDWICH

A savory and satisfying sandwich featuring grilled portobello mushrooms, perfect for a hearty lunch.

INGREDIENTS:	PREP TIME: 10 min	COOK TIME: 15 min	SERVINGS: 2 Servings

INGREDIENTS:	INSTRUCTIONS:
2 large portobello mushrooms, stems removed 2 Tbsp balsamic vinegar 2 Tbsp olive oil 1 clove garlic, minced Salt and pepper to taste 4 slices whole grain bread 1 avocado, sliced 1/2 cup arugula 1 small tomato, sliced	• In a small bowl, mix balsamic vinegar, olive oil, minced garlic, salt, and pepper. Brush the mixture onto the portobello mushrooms. • Preheat a grill or grill pan over medium heat. Grill the mushrooms for 5-7 minutes on each side until tender. • Toast the bread slices. • Assemble the sandwich by placing a grilled mushroom on a slice of bread, then topping with avocado slices, arugula, and tomato slices. Cover with another slice of bread. • Serve immediately.

NUTRITIONAL FACTS (per Serving): Calories: 340 | Total Fat: 22g | Saturated Fat: 3g | Fiber: 9g | Protein: 7g | Carbohydrate: 31g of which sugars: 6g | Vitamin A: 10% DV | Vitamin C: 20% DV | Calcium: 6% DV | Iron: 10% DV

CARROT AND GINGER SOUP

A warm and comforting soup made with fresh carrots and ginger, perfect for a light and healthy lunch.

INGREDIENTS:	PREP TIME: 10 min	COOK TIME: 25 min	SERVINGS: 2 Servings

INGREDIENTS:	INSTRUCTIONS:
1 Tbsp olive oil 1 small onion, diced 1 lb carrots, peeled and chopped 2 cloves garlic, minced 1 Tbsp fresh ginger, grated 3 cups vegetable broth Salt and pepper to taste 1/4 cup coconut milk (optional) Fresh cilantro for garnish	• In a large pot, heat olive oil over medium heat. Add diced onion and sauté until translucent, about 5 minutes. • Add carrots, garlic, and ginger, and cook for another 5 minutes. • Pour in the vegetable broth and bring to a boil. Reduce heat and simmer for 15-20 minutes, or until the carrots are tender. • Use an immersion blender to puree the soup until smooth. Alternatively, transfer the soup in batches to a blender and blend until smooth. • Stir in the coconut milk if using, and season with salt and pepper. • Garnish with fresh cilantro and serve hot.

NUTRITIONAL FACTS (per Serving): Calories: 180 | Total Fat: 7g | Saturated Fat: 2g | Fiber: 5g | Protein: 3g | Carbohydrate: 27g of which sugars: 12g | Vitamin A: 400% DV | Vitamin C: 15% DV | Calcium: 6% DV | Iron: 6% DV

VEGAN SUSHI ROLLS WITH AVOCADO AND CUCUMBER

Delicious and fresh vegan sushi rolls filled with creamy avocado and crisp cucumber, perfect for a light and healthy lunch.

INGREDIENTS:	PREP TIME: 20 min	COOK TIME: 10 min	SERVINGS: 2 Servings

INGREDIENTS	INSTRUCTIONS
1 cup sushi rice 1 1/4 cups water 2 Tbsp rice vinegar 1 Tbsp sugar 1/2 tsp salt 4 nori sheets 1 avocado, sliced 1/2 cucumber, julienned 1/4 cup carrots, julienned Soy sauce, for serving Pickled ginger, for serving (optional) Wasabi, for serving (optional)	**INSTRUCTIONS:** • Rinse sushi rice under cold water until the water runs clear. In a medium pot, combine rice and water. Bring to a boil, then reduce heat and simmer, covered, for 10 minutes. Remove from heat and let stand for 10 minutes. • In a small bowl, mix rice vinegar, sugar, and salt. Stir this mixture into the cooked rice. • Place a nori sheet on a bamboo sushi mat. Spread a thin layer of sushi rice over the nori, leaving a 1-inch border at the top. • Arrange avocado slices, cucumber, and carrots in a line along the bottom edge of the rice. • Roll the sushi tightly using the bamboo mat. Repeat with remaining nori sheets and fillings. • Slice each roll into 6-8 pieces and serve with soy sauce, pickled ginger, and wasabi.

NUTRITIONAL FACTS (per Serving): Calories: 300 | Total Fat: 10g | Saturated Fat: 1.5g | Fiber: 6g | Protein: 5g | Carbohydrate: 45g of which sugars: 4g | Vitamin A: 30% DV | Vitamin C: 15% DV | Calcium: 4% DV | Iron: 10% DV

SPAGHETTI SQUASH WITH MARINARA SAUCE

A delicious and low-carb alternative to traditional pasta, this spaghetti squash dish is served with a flavorful marinara sauce.

INGREDIENTS:	PREP TIME: 10 min	COOK TIME: 40 min	SERVINGS: 2 Servings

INGREDIENTS	INSTRUCTIONS
1 medium spaghetti squash 1 Tbsp olive oil Salt and pepper to taste 2 cups marinara sauce 1/4 cup fresh basil, chopped 1/4 cup grated Parmesan cheese (optional)	**INSTRUCTIONS:** • Preheat oven to 400°F (200°C). Cut the spaghetti squash in half lengthwise and scoop out the seeds. Drizzle with olive oil and season with salt and pepper. • Place the squash halves cut-side down on a baking sheet and roast for 30-40 minutes, or until tender. • While the squash is roasting, heat the marinara sauce in a saucepan over medium heat. • Remove the squash from the oven and use a fork to scrape out the strands of squash into a large bowl. • Divide the spaghetti squash between two plates and top with marinara sauce. Garnish with fresh basil and Parmesan cheese if desired. • Serve immediately.

NUTRITIONAL FACTS (per Serving): Calories: 180 | Total Fat: 8g | Saturated Fat: 1.5g | Fiber: 5g | Protein: 4g | Carbohydrate: 25g of which sugars: 10g | Vitamin A: 15% DV | Vitamin C: 20% DV | Calcium: 8% DV | Iron: 6% DV

BLACK BEAN AND CORN SALAD WITH LIME DRESSING

A refreshing and vibrant salad packed with protein and flavor, perfect for a light and healthy lunch.

INGREDIENTS:	PREP TIME: 10 min	COOK TIME: 0 min	SERVINGS: 2 Servings

INGREDIENTS:	INSTRUCTIONS:
1 cup black beans, cooked and drained	• In a large bowl, combine black beans, corn, red bell pepper, red onion, cilantro, and avocado.
1 cup corn kernels (fresh or frozen)	
1/2 red bell pepper, diced	• In a small bowl, whisk together olive oil, lime juice, garlic, ground cumin, salt, and pepper.
1/2 red onion, finely chopped	
1/4 cup fresh cilantro, chopped	• Pour the dressing over the salad and toss gently to combine.
1 avocado, diced	• Serve immediately or refrigerate until ready to eat.
2 Tbsp olive oil	
2 Tbsp lime juice	
1 clove garlic, minced	**NUTRITIONAL FACTS (per Serving):** Calories: 300 | Total Fat: 17g | Saturated Fat: 2.5g | Fiber: 12g | Protein: 7g | Carbohydrate: 34g of which sugars: 6g | Vitamin A: 20% DV | Vitamin C: 60% DV | Calcium: 8% DV | Iron: 15% DV
1/2 tsp ground cumin	
Salt and pepper to taste	

EGGPLANT AND LENTIL MOUSSAKA

A hearty and flavorful dish that combines eggplant, lentils, and a creamy topping, perfect for a comforting lunch.

INGREDIENTS:	PREP TIME: 20 min	COOK TIME: 40 min	SERVINGS: 2 Servings

INGREDIENTS:	INSTRUCTIONS:
1 large eggplant, sliced into rounds	• Preheat oven to 375°F (190°C). Brush eggplant slices with olive oil and place on a baking sheet. Roast for 20 minutes, flipping halfway through.
2 Tbsp olive oil	
1 cup cooked lentils	• In a skillet, sauté onion and garlic until translucent. Add cooked lentils, diced tomatoes, oregano, salt, and pepper. Cook for 5 minutes.
1 small onion, diced	
2 cloves garlic, minced	• In a small bowl, whisk together Greek yogurt, egg, and Parmesan cheese if using.
1 cup diced tomatoes	• In a baking dish, layer half of the roasted eggplant, then the lentil mixture, and top with the remaining eggplant. Spread the yogurt mixture over the top.
1 tsp dried oregano	
Salt and pepper to taste	• Bake for 20 minutes or until the top is golden and set.
1/2 cup plain Greek yogurt	• Serve hot.
1 egg	
1/4 cup grated Parmesan cheese (optional)	**NUTRITIONAL FACTS (per Serving):** Calories: 350 | Total Fat: 18g | Saturated Fat: 4.5g | Fiber: 12g | Protein: 15g | Carbohydrate: 38g of which sugars: 12g | Vitamin A: 15% DV | Vitamin C: 20% DV | Calcium: 15% DV | Iron: 20% DV

ROASTED BEET AND QUINOA SALAD

A nutritious and colorful salad featuring roasted beets and quinoa, perfect for a healthy lunch.

INGREDIENTS:	PREP TIME: 15 min	COOK TIME: 30 min	SERVINGS: 2 Servings
2 medium beets, roasted and diced	**INSTRUCTIONS:**		
1/2 cup quinoa, cooked	• Preheat oven to 400°F (200°C). Wrap beets in foil and roast for 30 minutes or until tender. Let cool, then peel and dice.		
1/2 cup arugula	• In a large bowl, combine roasted beets, cooked quinoa, arugula, feta cheese, walnuts, and red onion.		
1/4 cup feta cheese, crumbled (optional)			
1/4 cup walnuts, chopped	• In a small bowl, whisk together balsamic vinegar, olive oil, salt, and pepper.		
1/4 red onion, thinly sliced	• Drizzle the dressing over the salad and toss to combine.		
2 Tbsp balsamic vinegar	• Serve immediately or refrigerate until ready to eat.		
2 Tbsp olive oil	**NUTRITIONAL FACTS (per Serving):** Calories: 320 | Total Fat: 18g | Saturated Fat: 3.5g | Fiber: 7g | Protein: 9g | Carbohydrate: 33g of which sugars: 10g | Vitamin A: 15% DV | Vitamin C: 25% DV | Calcium: 15% DV | Iron: 20% DV		
Salt and pepper to taste			

HEARTY VEGETABLE AND BARLEY STEW

A comforting and filling stew packed with vegetables and barley, ideal for a nourishing lunch.

INGREDIENTS:	PREP TIME: 10 min	COOK TIME: 35 min	SERVINGS: 2 Servings
1 Tbsp olive oil	**INSTRUCTIONS:**		
1 small onion, diced			
2 cloves garlic, minced	• In a large pot, heat olive oil over medium heat. Add onion and garlic, and sauté until translucent, about 3 minutes.		
2 carrots, diced			
1 celery stalk, diced	• Add carrots, celery, and mushrooms, and cook for another 5 minutes until vegetables are softened.		
1 cup mushrooms, sliced			
1/2 cup barley	• Stir in barley, vegetable broth, diced tomatoes, thyme, rosemary, salt, and pepper. Bring to a boil.		
4 cups vegetable broth			
1 can (14.5 oz) diced tomatoes	• Reduce heat and simmer for 25 minutes until barley is tender.		
1 tsp dried thyme	• Add chopped kale and cook for an additional 5 minutes until wilted.		
1 tsp dried rosemary	• Serve hot.		
Salt and pepper to taste	**NUTRITIONAL FACTS (per Serving):** Calories: 280 | Total Fat: 7g | Saturated Fat: 1g | Fiber: 10g | Protein: 7g | Carbohydrate: 46g of which sugars: 10g | Vitamin A: 120% DV | Vitamin C: 60% DV | Calcium: 10% DV | Iron: 20% DV		
2 cups kale, chopped			

4. AFTERNOON SNACKS

AVOCADO AND TOMATO SALSA WITH WHOLE-GRAIN CRACKERS

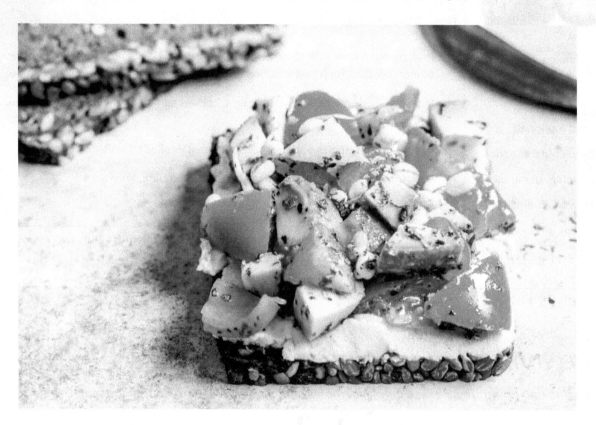

A refreshing and zesty salsa paired with crunchy whole-grain crackers, perfect for a healthy afternoon snack.

INGREDIENTS:	PREP TIME: 10 min	COOK TIME: 0 min	SERVINGS: 2 Servings

INGREDIENTS:	
1 avocado, diced	**INSTRUCTIONS:**
1 cup cherry tomatoes, diced	• In a bowl, combine diced avocado, cherry tomatoes, red onion, jalapeño, cilantro, lime juice, salt, and pepper.
1/4 red onion, finely chopped	• Mix gently to combine.
1/2 jalapeño, seeded and minced	• Serve the salsa with whole-grain crackers.
2 Tbsp fresh cilantro, chopped	
1 Tbsp lime juice	
Salt and pepper to taste	**NUTRITIONAL FACTS (per Serving):** Calories: 200 | Total Fat: 12g | Saturated Fat: 1.5g | Fiber: 6g | Protein: 3g | Carbohydrate: 22g of which sugars: 3g | Vitamin A: 15% DV | Vitamin C: 25% DV | Calcium: 4% DV | Iron: 6% DV
12 whole-grain crackers	

ALMOND AND CRANBERRY TRAIL MIX

A nutritious and easy-to-make trail mix perfect for a mid-morning energy boost.

INGREDIENTS:	PREP TIME: 5 min	COOK TIME: 0 min	SERVINGS: 2 Servings
1/4 cup almonds 1/4 cup dried cranberries 1/4 cup pumpkin seeds 1/4 cup sunflower seeds 2 Tbsp dark chocolate chips (optional)	**INSTRUCTIONS:** • In a bowl, combine almonds, dried cranberries, pumpkin seeds, sunflower seeds, and dark chocolate chips if using. • Mix well and divide into two servings. • Store in an airtight container until ready to eat. **NUTRITIONAL FACTS (per Serving):** Calories: 200 | Total Fat: 12g | Saturated Fat: 2g | Fiber: 4g | Protein: 6g | Carbohydrate: 20g of which sugars: 12g | Calcium: 4% DV | Iron: 10% DV | Vitamin E: 20% DV		

SPICED CHICKPEA SNACK

A crunchy and flavorful snack made with roasted chickpeas, perfect for a nutritious afternoon pick-me-up.

INGREDIENTS:	PREP TIME: 5 min	COOK TIME: 30 min	SERVINGS: 2 Servings
1 cup chickpeas, cooked and drained 1 Tbsp olive oil 1/2 tsp smoked paprika 1/2 tsp ground cumin 1/4 tsp cayenne pepper (optional) 1/2 tsp sea salt	**INSTRUCTIONS:** • Preheat oven to 400°F (200°C). • In a bowl, toss chickpeas with olive oil, smoked paprika, ground cumin, cayenne pepper (if using), and sea salt. • Spread the chickpeas in a single layer on a baking sheet. • Roast for 25-30 minutes, or until crispy, stirring halfway through. • Allow to cool slightly before serving. **NUTRITIONAL FACTS (per Serving):** Calories: 180 | Total Fat: 8g | Saturated Fat: 1g | Fiber: 7g | Protein: 6g | Carbohydrate: 20g of which sugars: 1g | Vitamin A: 8% DV | Vitamin C: 2% DV | Calcium: 4% DV | Iron: 10% DV		

ROASTED GARLIC AND HERB CASHEWS

These savory and crunchy cashews are perfect for a satisfying afternoon snack, packed with flavor from garlic and herbs.

INGREDIENTS:	PREP TIME: 5 min	COOK TIME: 15 min	SERVINGS: 2 Servings
1 cup raw cashews 1 Tbsp olive oil 1/2 tsp garlic powder 1/2 tsp dried rosemary 1/2 tsp dried thyme 1/4 tsp sea salt 1/4 tsp black pepper	**INSTRUCTIONS:** • Preheat oven to 350°F (175°C). Line a baking sheet with parchment paper. • In a bowl, toss cashews with olive oil, garlic powder, dried rosemary, dried thyme, sea salt, and black pepper. • Spread the cashews in a single layer on the prepared baking sheet. • Roast for 12-15 minutes, stirring halfway through, until golden brown and fragrant. • Allow to cool before serving.		
	NUTRITIONAL FACTS (per Serving): Calories: 220 | Total Fat: 18g | Saturated Fat: 3g | Fiber: 2g | Protein: 6g | Carbohydrate: 12g of which sugars: 2g | Vitamin A: 0% DV | Vitamin C: 0% DV | Calcium: 2% DV | Iron: 10% DV		

FRESH MANGO AND LIME SALAD

A refreshing and tangy salad featuring sweet mango and zesty lime, perfect for a light and healthy snack.

INGREDIENTS:	PREP TIME: 10 min	COOK TIME: 0 min	SERVINGS: 2 Servings
2 ripe mangoes, peeled and diced 2 Tbsp lime juice 1 Tbsp fresh mint, chopped 1/4 tsp chili powder (optional) Pinch of sea salt	**INSTRUCTIONS:** • In a bowl, combine diced mangoes, lime juice, fresh mint, chili powder (if using), and a pinch of sea salt. • Toss gently to mix all ingredients. • Serve immediately or chill in the refrigerator until ready to eat.		
	NUTRITIONAL FACTS (per Serving): Calories: 120 | Total Fat: 0.5g | Saturated Fat: 0g | Fiber: 3g | Protein: 1g | Carbohydrate: 30g of which sugars: 24g | Vitamin A: 35% DV | Vitamin C: 100% DV | Calcium: 2% DV | Iron: 2% DV		

CELERY STICKS WITH SUNFLOWER SEED BUTTER

A simple and nutritious snack combining crunchy celery sticks with creamy sunflower seed butter.

INGREDIENTS:	PREP TIME: 5 min	COOK TIME: 0 min	SERVINGS: 2 Servings
4 celery stalks, cut into sticks 4 Tbsp sunflower seed butter	**INSTRUCTIONS:** • Wash and cut celery stalks into sticks. • Serve each serving with 2 Tbsp of sunflower seed butter for dipping. **NUTRITIONAL FACTS (per Serving):** Calories: 200 | Total Fat: 16g | Saturated Fat: 2g | Fiber: 4g | Protein: 7g | Carbohydrate: 9g of which sugars: 3g | Vitamin A: 10% DV | Vitamin C: 15% DV | Calcium: 4% DV | Iron: 8% DV		

TURMERIC-SPICED POPCORN

A healthy and flavorful snack, this turmeric-spiced popcorn is perfect for an afternoon treat.

INGREDIENTS:	PREP TIME: 5 min	COOK TIME: 10 min	SERVINGS: 2 Servings
1/4 cup popcorn kernels 1 Tbsp coconut oil 1/2 tsp ground turmeric 1/4 tsp ground cumin 1/4 tsp sea salt	**INSTRUCTIONS:** • In a large pot, heat coconut oil over medium heat. Add popcorn kernels and cover with a lid. • Shake the pot occasionally until popping slows to about 2-3 seconds between pops. • Remove from heat and transfer popcorn to a large bowl. • Sprinkle with ground turmeric, ground cumin, and sea salt. Toss to coat evenly. • Serve immediately. **NUTRITIONAL FACTS (per Serving):** Calories: 140 | Total Fat: 7g | Saturated Fat: 5g | Fiber: 3g | Protein: 2g | Carbohydrate: 18g of which sugars: 0g | Vitamin A: 2% DV | Vitamin C: 0% DV | Calcium: 1% DV | Iron: 3% DV		

VEGAN CHEESE AND CUCUMBER SLICES

A refreshing and savory snack pairing vegan cheese with crisp cucumber slices.

INGREDIENTS:	PREP TIME: 5 min	COOK TIME: 0 min	SERVINGS: 2 Servings
1 cucumber, sliced into rounds 1/4 cup vegan cheese, sliced or spreadable	**INSTRUCTIONS:** • Wash and slice the cucumber into rounds. • Spread or place a small amount of vegan cheese on each cucumber slice. • Arrange on a plate and serve immediately. **NUTRITIONAL FACTS (per Serving):** Calories: 80 | Total Fat: 4g | Saturated Fat: 1g | Fiber: 2g | Protein: 2g | Carbohydrate: 10g of which sugars: 2g | Vitamin A: 4% DV | Vitamin C: 10% DV | Calcium: 4% DV | Iron: 2% DV		

BAKED APPLE CHIPS WITH CINNAMON

Crispy and sweet, these baked apple chips with cinnamon make a delightful afternoon snack.

INGREDIENTS:	PREP TIME: 10 min	COOK TIME: 2 h	SERVINGS: 2 Servings
2 apples, thinly sliced 1 tsp ground cinnamon	**INSTRUCTIONS:** • Preheat oven to 225°F (110°C). Line a baking sheet with parchment paper. • Arrange apple slices in a single layer on the prepared baking sheet. • Sprinkle ground cinnamon evenly over the apple slices. • Bake for 2 hours, turning the slices halfway through, until crisp. • Allow to cool before serving. **NUTRITIONAL FACTS (per Serving):** Calories: 70 | Total Fat: 0g | Saturated Fat: 0g | Fiber: 4g | Protein: 0g | Carbohydrate: 18g of which sugars: 14g | Vitamin A: 2% DV | Vitamin C: 8% DV | Calcium: 2% DV | Iron: 2% DV		

5. DINNER

MUSHROOM AND SPINACH RISOTTO

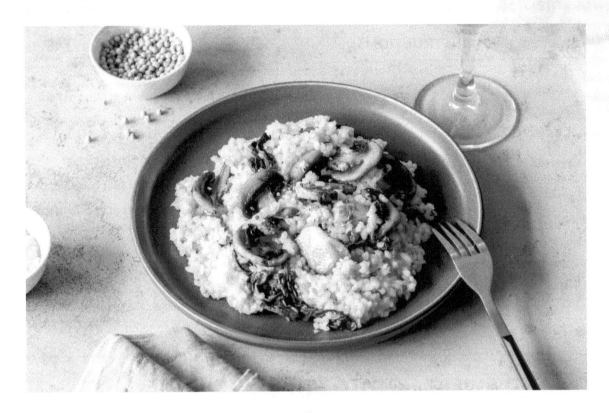

A creamy and flavorful risotto featuring mushrooms and spinach, perfect for a comforting dinner.

INGREDIENTS:	PREP TIME: 10 min	COOK TIME: 30 min	SERVINGS: 2 Servings
1 Tbsp olive oil 1 small onion, finely chopped 2 cloves garlic, minced 1 cup Arborio rice 1/2 cup white wine (optional) 3 cups vegetable broth, warmed 1 cup mushrooms, sliced 2 cups fresh spinach, chopped 1/4 cup nutritional yeast (optional) Salt and pepper to taste Fresh parsley for garnish	**INSTRUCTIONS:** • Heat olive oil in a large pan over medium heat. Add onion and garlic, and sauté until translucent, about 3 minutes. • Stir in Arborio rice and cook for 2 minutes until lightly toasted. • Pour in white wine (if using) and stir until absorbed. • Add warm vegetable broth, one cup at a time, stirring frequently until the liquid is absorbed before adding more. • In a separate pan, sauté mushrooms until browned, then add to the risotto. • When the rice is creamy and cooked, stir in chopped spinach until wilted. • Add nutritional yeast (if using), salt, and pepper. Stir well. • Garnish with fresh parsley and serve.		
	NUTRITIONAL FACTS (per Serving): Calories: 380 | Total Fat: 8g | Saturated Fat: 1.5g | Fiber: 5g | Protein: 10g | Carbohydrate: 64g of which sugars: 4g | Vitamin A: 50% DV | Vitamin C: 25% DV | Calcium: 6% DV | Iron: 20% DV		

BAKED EGGPLANT PARMESAN

A healthy twist on the classic dish, this baked eggplant Parmesan is both delicious and nutritious.

INGREDIENTS:	PREP TIME: 20 min	COOK TIME: 40 min	SERVINGS: 2 Servings

INGREDIENTS:	INSTRUCTIONS:
1 large eggplant, sliced into rounds 1 cup marinara sauce 1/2 cup whole wheat breadcrumbs 1/4 cup grated Parmesan cheese 1/4 cup mozzarella cheese, shredded (optional) 1 egg, beaten 2 Tbsp olive oil 1/2 tsp dried oregano Salt and pepper to taste Fresh basil leaves for garnish	• Preheat oven to 375°F (190°C). Line a baking sheet with parchment paper. • Sprinkle eggplant slices with salt and let sit for 10 minutes. Rinse and pat dry. • Dip each eggplant slice in the beaten egg, then coat with breadcrumbs mixed with Parmesan cheese, dried oregano, salt, and pepper. • Place eggplant slices on the baking sheet and drizzle with olive oil. • Bake for 20 minutes, flip, then bake for another 20 minutes until golden and crispy. • Spread a layer of marinara sauce in a baking dish, add a layer of eggplant, top with more sauce and cheese. • Bake for 10-15 minutes until cheese is melted and bubbly. • Garnish with fresh basil leaves and serve.

NUTRITIONAL FACTS (per Serving): Calories: 320 | Total Fat: 18g | Saturated Fat: 4.5g | Fiber: 7g | Protein: 11g | Carbohydrate: 32g of which sugars: 10g | Vitamin A: 10% DV | Vitamin C: 15% DV | Calcium: 20% DV | Iron: 8% DV

LENTIL AND SWEET POTATO SHEPHERD'S PIE

A hearty and comforting dish made with lentils and sweet potatoes, perfect for a nourishing dinner.

INGREDIENTS:	PREP TIME: 20 min	COOK TIME: 45 min	SERVINGS: 2 Servings

INGREDIENTS:	INSTRUCTIONS:
1 cup green lentils, cooked and drained 1 large sweet potato, peeled and diced 1 small onion, diced 2 cloves garlic, minced 1 carrot, diced 1 celery stalk, diced 1 cup vegetable broth 1 Tbsp olive oil 1 tsp dried thyme 1 tsp dried rosemary Salt and pepper to taste 1/4 cup almond milk 1 Tbsp nutritional yeast (optional)	• Preheat oven to 375°F (190°C). • In a large pot, boil sweet potatoes until tender, about 15 minutes. Drain and mash with almond milk and nutritional yeast if using. Season with salt and pepper. • In a skillet, heat olive oil over medium heat. Add onion, garlic, carrot, and celery. Sauté until softened, about 5 minutes. • Add cooked lentils, vegetable broth, dried thyme, dried rosemary, salt, and pepper. Simmer for 10 minutes until the mixture thickens. • Transfer the lentil mixture to a baking dish. Spread mashed sweet potatoes on top. • Bake for 20 minutes until the top is golden brown. • Serve hot.

NUTRITIONAL FACTS (per Serving): Calories: 400 | Total Fat: 10g | Saturated Fat: 1.5g | Fiber: 15g | Protein: 15g | Carbohydrate: 65g of which sugars: 15g | Vitamin A: 400% DV | Vitamin C: 35% DV | Calcium: 10% DV | Iron: 25% DV

QUINOA-STUFFED BELL PEPPERS

These colorful bell peppers are stuffed with a savory quinoa mixture, making for a healthy and delicious dinner option.

INGREDIENTS:	PREP TIME: 15 min	COOK TIME: 30 min	SERVINGS: 2 Servings

INGREDIENTS:	INSTRUCTIONS:
2 large bell peppers, halved and seeded	
1/2 cup quinoa, cooked	• Preheat oven to 375°F (190°C).
1/2 cup black beans, cooked and drained	• In a large bowl, combine cooked quinoa, black beans, corn, diced tomatoes, red onion, ground cumin, chili powder, cilantro, olive oil, salt, and pepper.
1/4 cup corn kernels (fresh or frozen)	• Stuff each bell pepper half with the quinoa mixture.
1/4 cup diced tomatoes	• Place the stuffed peppers in a baking dish and cover with foil.
1/4 cup red onion, diced	• Bake for 25-30 minutes, or until the peppers are tender.
1 tsp ground cumin	• Serve warm.
1/2 tsp chili powder	
2 Tbsp fresh cilantro, chopped	**NUTRITIONAL FACTS (per Serving):** Calories: 300 | Total Fat: 12g | Saturated Fat: 1.5g |
2 Tbsp olive oil	Fiber: 10g | Protein: 8g | Carbohydrate: 40g of which sugars: 6g | Vitamin A: 80% DV |
Salt and pepper to taste	Vitamin C: 220% DV | Calcium: 6% DV | Iron: 15% DV

VEGAN PAD THAI WITH TOFU

A plant-based version of the classic Thai dish, featuring tofu and a flavorful sauce over noodles.

INGREDIENTS:	PREP TIME: 20 min	COOK TIME: 15 min	SERVINGS: 2 Servings

INGREDIENTS:	INSTRUCTIONS:
4 oz rice noodles	
1 block (8 oz) firm tofu, drained and cubed	• Cook rice noodles according to package instructions. Drain and set aside.
1 cup bean sprouts	• In a small bowl, whisk together tamari, lime juice, peanut butter, maple syrup, and chili garlic sauce to make the sauce.
1/2 cup shredded carrots	
1/2 cup red bell pepper, sliced	• In a large skillet, heat peanut oil over medium heat. Add tofu cubes and cook until golden brown on all sides, about 5-7 minutes. Remove tofu from the skillet and set aside.
2 green onions, chopped	
2 cloves garlic, minced	• In the same skillet, add garlic, bean sprouts, shredded carrots, red bell pepper, and green onions. Sauté for 5 minutes until vegetables are tender.
2 Tbsp peanut oil	
3 Tbsp tamari or soy sauce	• Add cooked noodles, tofu, and sauce to the skillet. Toss to combine and heat through.
2 Tbsp lime juice	
1 Tbsp peanut butter	• Serve immediately, garnished with crushed peanuts, fresh cilantro, and lime wedges.
1 Tbsp maple syrup	
1 tsp chili garlic sauce (optional)	
1/4 cup crushed peanuts	**NUTRITIONAL FACTS (per Serving):** Calories: 420 | Total Fat: 20g | Saturated Fat: 3g | Fiber:
2 Tbsp fresh cilantro, chopped	6g | Protein: 16g | Carbohydrate: 48g of which sugars: 8g | Vitamin A: 70% DV | Vitamin C:
Lime wedges	60% DV | Calcium: 15% DV | Iron: 20% DV

SPINACH AND CHICKPEA CURRY

A flavorful and nutritious curry featuring spinach and chickpeas, perfect for a comforting dinner.

INGREDIENTS:	PREP TIME: 10 min	COOK TIME: 25 min	SERVINGS: 2 Servings

INGREDIENTS:	INSTRUCTIONS:
1 Tbsp olive oil 1 small onion, diced 2 cloves garlic, minced 1 tsp grated ginger 1 can (14.5 oz) diced tomatoes 1 can (14.5 oz) chickpeas, drained and rinsed 4 cups fresh spinach 1 tsp ground cumin 1 tsp ground coriander 1/2 tsp turmeric 1/2 tsp chili powder Salt and pepper to taste 1/4 cup coconut milk Fresh cilantro for garnish	• Heat olive oil in a large pot over medium heat. Add onion, garlic, and ginger, and sauté until softened, about 5 minutes. • Stir in cumin, coriander, turmeric, and chili powder. Cook for 1 minute until fragrant. • Add diced tomatoes and chickpeas. Simmer for 10 minutes. • Add spinach and cook until wilted, about 5 minutes. • Stir in coconut milk and season with salt and pepper. • Serve hot, garnished with fresh cilantro.

NUTRITIONAL FACTS (per Serving): Calories: 280 | Total Fat: 10g | Saturated Fat: 4g | Fiber: 12g | Protein: 10g | Carbohydrate: 36g of which sugars: 8g | Vitamin A: 150% DV | Vitamin C: 70% DV | Calcium: 15% DV | Iron: 30% DV

VEGAN LASAGNA WITH CASHEW CHEESE

A delicious and hearty vegan lasagna layered with cashew cheese and vegetables, perfect for a satisfying dinner.

INGREDIENTS:	PREP TIME: 30 min	COOK TIME: 45 min	SERVINGS: 2 Servings

INGREDIENTS:	INSTRUCTIONS:
6 lasagna noodles 2 cups marinara sauce 1 zucchini, thinly sliced 1 cup spinach, chopped 1/2 cup mushrooms, sliced 1 cup cashews, soaked in water for 4 hours 1/4 cup water 2 Tbsp nutritional yeast 1 Tbsp lemon juice 1 clove garlic, minced Salt and pepper to taste	• Preheat oven to 375°F (190°C). Cook lasagna noodles according to package instructions. • Drain and rinse cashews. In a blender, combine cashews, water, nutritional yeast, lemon juice, garlic, salt, and pepper. Blend until smooth. • In a baking dish, spread a layer of marinara sauce. Place a layer of lasagna noodles on top. • Spread a layer of cashew cheese over the noodles, followed by a layer of zucchini, spinach, and mushrooms. • Repeat layers until all ingredients are used, finishing with a layer of marinara sauce. • Cover with foil and bake for 30 minutes. Remove foil and bake for an additional 15 minutes until bubbly and golden. • Let sit for 10 minutes before serving.

NUTRITIONAL FACTS (per Serving): Calories: 450 | Total Fat: 20g | Saturated Fat: 3g | Fiber: 8g | Protein: 14g | Carbohydrate: 58g of which sugars: 10g | Vitamin A: 40% DV | Vitamin C: 30% DV | Calcium: 10% DV | Iron: 25% DV

STUFFED ACORN SQUASH WITH WILD RICE

A flavorful and satisfying dish featuring acorn squash stuffed with a savory wild rice mixture, perfect for a nourishing dinner.

INGREDIENTS:	PREP TIME: 15 min	COOK TIME: 45 min	SERVINGS: 2 Servings

INGREDIENTS:	INSTRUCTIONS:
1 acorn squash, halved and seeded 1/2 cup wild rice, cooked 1/4 cup dried cranberries 1/4 cup chopped pecans 1/4 cup celery, diced 1/4 cup onion, diced 1 Tbsp olive oil 1 tsp dried thyme Salt and pepper to taste	• Preheat oven to 400°F (200°C). Place acorn squash halves cut side down on a baking sheet. Roast for 30 minutes until tender. • In a skillet, heat olive oil over medium heat. Add celery and onion, and sauté until softened, about 5 minutes. • In a bowl, combine cooked wild rice, dried cranberries, chopped pecans, sautéed celery, onion, dried thyme, salt, and pepper. • Fill each acorn squash half with the wild rice mixture. • Return to the oven and bake for an additional 15 minutes. • Serve warm.

NUTRITIONAL FACTS (per Serving): Calories: 350 | Total Fat: 14g | Saturated Fat: 2g | Fiber: 8g | Protein: 5g | Carbohydrate: 54g of which sugars: 14g | Vitamin A: 20% DV | Vitamin C: 30% DV | Calcium: 8% DV | Iron: 10% DV

MOROCCAN VEGETABLE TAGINE

A vibrant and aromatic vegetable stew, rich with Moroccan spices, perfect for a comforting dinner.

INGREDIENTS:	PREP TIME: 15 min	COOK TIME: 40 min	SERVINGS: 2 Servings

INGREDIENTS:	INSTRUCTIONS:
1 Tbsp olive oil 1 small onion, diced 2 cloves garlic, minced 1 carrot, sliced 1 zucchini, sliced 1 red bell pepper, diced 1 cup chickpeas, cooked and drained 1 can (14.5 oz) diced tomatoes 1/2 cup vegetable broth 1 tsp ground cumin 1 tsp ground coriander 1/2 tsp ground cinnamon 1/4 tsp ground ginger 1/4 tsp ground turmeric Salt and pepper to taste 1/4 cup fresh cilantro, chopped 1/4 cup slivered almonds, toasted	• In a large pot, heat olive oil over medium heat. Add onion and garlic, and sauté until fragrant, about 3 minutes. • Add carrot, zucchini, and red bell pepper. Cook for 5 minutes until vegetables begin to soften. • Stir in chickpeas, diced tomatoes, vegetable broth, ground cumin, ground coriander, ground cinnamon, ground ginger, ground turmeric, salt, and pepper. • Bring to a boil, then reduce heat and simmer for 25 minutes until vegetables are tender and flavors are well combined. • Garnish with fresh cilantro and toasted almonds before serving.

NUTRITIONAL FACTS (per Serving): Calories: 300 | Total Fat: 12g | Saturated Fat: 1.5g | Fiber: 10g | Protein: 8g | Carbohydrate: 42g of which sugars: 12g | Vitamin A: 120% DV | Vitamin C: 100% DV | Calcium: 10% DV | Iron: 15% DV

CREAMY COCONUT LENTIL CURRY

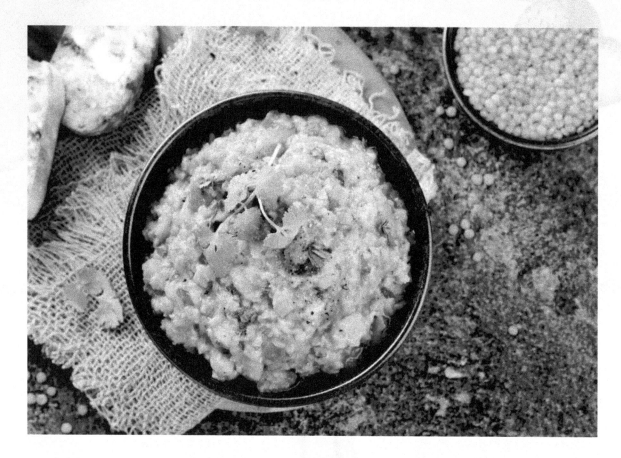

This creamy and flavorful curry is made with lentils and coconut milk, creating a rich and comforting dinner.

INGREDIENTS:	PREP TIME: 10 min	COOK TIME: 30 min	SERVINGS: 2 Servings

INGREDIENTS	INSTRUCTIONS
1 Tbsp coconut oil 1 small onion, diced 2 cloves garlic, minced 1 Tbsp fresh ginger, minced 1 cup red lentils, rinsed 1 can (14.5 oz) diced tomatoes 1 can (14 oz) coconut milk 1 cup vegetable broth 1 Tbsp curry powder 1 tsp ground cumin 1/2 tsp ground turmeric Salt and pepper to taste Fresh cilantro for garnish	**INSTRUCTIONS:** • Heat coconut oil in a large pot over medium heat. Add onion, garlic, and ginger, and sauté until fragrant, about 3 minutes. • Stir in curry powder, ground cumin, and ground turmeric. Cook for 1 minute until fragrant. • Add red lentils, diced tomatoes, coconut milk, and vegetable broth. Bring to a boil, then reduce heat and simmer for 25-30 minutes until lentils are tender and the curry has thickened. • Season with salt and pepper. • Serve hot, garnished with fresh cilantro.

NUTRITIONAL FACTS (per Serving): Calories: 420 | Total Fat: 24g | Saturated Fat: 20g | Fiber: 12g | Protein: 14g | Carbohydrate: 40g of which sugars: 8g | Vitamin A: 15% DV | Vitamin C: 20% DV | Calcium: 6% DV | Iron: 30% DV

BLACK BEAN AND BUTTERNUT SQUASH CHILI

A hearty and flavorful chili that combines black beans and butternut squash for a nutritious and satisfying dinner.

INGREDIENTS:	PREP TIME: 10 min	COOK TIME: 40 min	SERVINGS: 2 Servings

INGREDIENTS:	INSTRUCTIONS:
1 Tbsp olive oil 1 small onion, diced 2 cloves garlic, minced 1 small butternut squash, peeled and diced 1 can (14.5 oz) black beans, drained and rinsed 1 can (14.5 oz) diced tomatoes 1 cup vegetable broth 1 tsp ground cumin 1 tsp chili powder 1/2 tsp smoked paprika Salt and pepper to taste 1/4 cup fresh cilantro, chopped (optional)	• In a large pot, heat olive oil over medium heat. Add onion and garlic, and sauté until fragrant, about 3 minutes. • Add diced butternut squash and cook for 5 minutes. • Stir in black beans, diced tomatoes, vegetable broth, ground cumin, chili powder, smoked paprika, salt, and pepper. • Bring to a boil, then reduce heat and simmer for 30 minutes, or until the squash is tender. • Serve hot, garnished with fresh cilantro if desired.
	NUTRITIONAL FACTS (per Serving): Calories: 350 | Total Fat: 8g | Saturated Fat: 1g | Fiber: 14g | Protein: 12g | Carbohydrate: 62g of which sugars: 12g | Vitamin A: 300% DV | Vitamin C: 60% DV | Calcium: 15% DV | Iron: 20% DV

ROASTED CAULIFLOWER AND CHICKPEAS WITH TAHINI SAUCE

A delicious and hearty dish featuring roasted cauliflower and chickpeas, drizzled with a creamy tahini sauce.

INGREDIENTS:	PREP TIME: 10 min	COOK TIME: 30 min	SERVINGS: 2 Servings

INGREDIENTS:	INSTRUCTIONS:
1 small cauliflower, cut into florets 1 can (14.5 oz) chickpeas, drained and rinsed 2 Tbsp olive oil 1 tsp ground cumin 1/2 tsp smoked paprika Salt and pepper to taste 2 Tbsp tahini 1 Tbsp lemon juice 1 Tbsp water 1 clove garlic, minced Salt and pepper to taste	• Preheat oven to 400°F (200°C). Line a baking sheet with parchment paper. • In a large bowl, toss cauliflower florets and chickpeas with olive oil, ground cumin, smoked paprika, salt, and pepper. • Spread the mixture on the baking sheet and roast for 25-30 minutes until the cauliflower is tender and golden. • In a small bowl, whisk together tahini, lemon juice, water, garlic, salt, and pepper to make the sauce. • Serve the roasted cauliflower and chickpeas drizzled with tahini sauce.
	NUTRITIONAL FACTS (per Serving): Calories: 320 | Total Fat: 18g | Saturated Fat: 2.5g | Fiber: 10g | Protein: 10g | Carbohydrate: 34g of which sugars: 6g | Vitamin A: 10% DV | Vitamin C: 100% DV | Calcium: 10% DV | Iron: 20% DV

ZUCCHINI AND TOMATO GRATIN

A delicious and light zucchini and tomato gratin, perfect for a healthy and flavorful dinner.

INGREDIENTS:	PREP TIME: 15 min	COOK TIME: 25 min	SERVINGS: 2 Servings

INGREDIENTS:	INSTRUCTIONS:
2 medium zucchinis, thinly sliced 2 medium tomatoes, thinly sliced 1/4 cup breadcrumbs 1/4 cup grated Parmesan cheese 1 Tbsp olive oil 2 cloves garlic, minced 1 tsp dried oregano Salt and pepper to taste Fresh basil leaves for garnish	• Preheat oven to 375°F (190°C). Lightly grease a baking dish with olive oil. • Layer the zucchini and tomato slices in the baking dish, alternating them. • In a small bowl, combine breadcrumbs, grated Parmesan cheese, minced garlic, dried oregano, salt, and pepper. • Sprinkle the breadcrumb mixture evenly over the vegetables. Drizzle with olive oil. • Bake for 25 minutes, or until the vegetables are tender and the top is golden brown. • Garnish with fresh basil leaves and serve hot.
	NUTRITIONAL FACTS (per Serving): Calories: 220 | Total Fat: 10g | Saturated Fat: 2.5g | Fiber: 4g | Protein: 8g | Carbohydrate: 26g of which sugars: 8g | Vitamin A: 25% DV | Vitamin C: 50% DV | Calcium: 15% DV | Iron: 10% DV

BAKED TOFU WITH STIR-FRIED VEGETABLES

A delicious and nutritious dinner featuring crispy baked tofu and a colorful medley of stir-fried vegetables.

INGREDIENTS:	PREP TIME: 15 min	COOK TIME: 30 min	SERVINGS: 2 Servings

INGREDIENTS:	INSTRUCTIONS:
1 block (8 oz) firm tofu, drained and cubed 2 Tbsp soy sauce or tamari 1 Tbsp olive oil 1 cup broccoli florets 1 red bell pepper, sliced 1 carrot, julienned 1/2 cup snap peas 2 cloves garlic, minced 1 Tbsp fresh ginger, minced 2 Tbsp sesame oil 1 Tbsp sesame seeds Salt and pepper to taste	• Preheat oven to 400°F (200°C). Toss tofu cubes with soy sauce and olive oil. Spread on a baking sheet and bake for 25 minutes, flipping halfway through. • In a large skillet, heat sesame oil over medium heat. Add garlic and ginger, and sauté for 1 minute. • Add broccoli, bell pepper, carrot, and snap peas to the skillet. Stir-fry for 5-7 minutes until vegetables are tender-crisp. • Add baked tofu to the skillet and toss to combine. Season with salt and pepper. • Garnish with sesame seeds and serve hot.
	NUTRITIONAL FACTS (per Serving): Calories: 320 | Total Fat: 18g | Saturated Fat: 2.5g | Fiber: 8g | Protein: 15g | Carbohydrate: 24g of which sugars: 6g | Vitamin A: 90% DV | Vitamin C: 150% DV | Calcium: 20% DV | Iron: 20% DV

CAULIFLOWER AND POTATO CURRY

A flavorful and comforting curry made with tender cauliflower and potatoes, perfect for a satisfying dinner.

INGREDIENTS:	PREP TIME: 10 min	COOK TIME: 30 min	SERVINGS: 2 Servings

INGREDIENTS:	INSTRUCTIONS:
1 Tbsp olive oil 1 small onion, diced 2 cloves garlic, minced 1 Tbsp fresh ginger, minced 1 Tbsp curry powder 1/2 tsp ground cumin 1/2 tsp ground turmeric 1/4 tsp cayenne pepper (optional) 1 cup cauliflower florets 2 medium potatoes, diced 1 can (14.5 oz) diced tomatoes 1 cup coconut milk Salt and pepper to taste Fresh cilantro for garnish	• Heat olive oil in a large pot over medium heat. Add onion, garlic, and ginger, and sauté until fragrant, about 3 minutes. • Stir in curry powder, ground cumin, ground turmeric, and cayenne pepper (if using). Cook for 1 minute until fragrant. • Add cauliflower florets and diced potatoes, and stir to coat with spices. • Pour in diced tomatoes and coconut milk. Bring to a boil, then reduce heat and simmer for 20-25 minutes until vegetables are tender. • Season with salt and pepper. Serve hot, garnished with fresh cilantro.

NUTRITIONAL FACTS (per Serving): Calories: 380 | Total Fat: 20g | Saturated Fat: 10g | Fiber: 9g | Protein: 7g | Carbohydrate: 45g of which sugars: 10g | Vitamin A: 10% DV | Vitamin C: 80% DV | Calcium: 8% DV | Iron: 20% DV

MEDITERRANEAN QUINOA BOWLS

These vibrant and nutritious quinoa bowls are packed with Mediterranean flavors, perfect for a wholesome dinner.

INGREDIENTS:	PREP TIME: 15 min	COOK TIME: 20 min	SERVINGS: 2 Servings

INGREDIENTS:	INSTRUCTIONS:
1 cup quinoa, cooked 1/2 cup cherry tomatoes, halved 1/2 cucumber, diced 1/4 cup Kalamata olives, pitted and sliced 1/4 cup red onion, finely chopped 1/4 cup feta cheese, crumbled (optional) 2 Tbsp fresh parsley, chopped 2 Tbsp olive oil 1 Tbsp lemon juice 1 tsp dried oregano Salt and pepper to taste	• In a large bowl, combine cooked quinoa, cherry tomatoes, cucumber, Kalamata olives, red onion, feta cheese (if using), and fresh parsley. • In a small bowl, whisk together olive oil, lemon juice, dried oregano, salt, and pepper. • Pour the dressing over the quinoa mixture and toss to combine. • Serve immediately or refrigerate until ready to eat.

NUTRITIONAL FACTS (per Serving): Calories: 320 | Total Fat: 18g | Saturated Fat: 4g | Fiber: 6g | Protein: 9g | Carbohydrate: 33g of which sugars: 4g | Vitamin A: 15% DV | Vitamin C: 25% DV | Calcium: 10% DV | Iron: 15% DV

VEGAN MEATLOAF WITH LENTILS AND OATS

A hearty and flavorful vegan meatloaf made with lentils and oats, perfect for a comforting dinner.

INGREDIENTS:	PREP TIME: 15 min	COOK TIME: 45 min	SERVINGS: 2 Servings

INGREDIENTS	INSTRUCTIONS:
1 cup cooked lentils 1/2 cup rolled oats 1 small onion, finely chopped 2 cloves garlic, minced 1/4 cup carrots, grated 1/4 cup celery, finely chopped 2 Tbsp ground flaxseed mixed with 5 Tbsp water (flax egg) 2 Tbsp tomato paste 1 Tbsp soy sauce or tamari 1 tsp dried thyme 1 tsp dried oregano Salt and pepper to taste	• Preheat oven to 375°F (190°C). Line a loaf pan with parchment paper. • In a large bowl, combine cooked lentils, rolled oats, chopped onion, minced garlic, grated carrots, and chopped celery. • Add the flax egg, tomato paste, soy sauce, dried thyme, dried oregano, salt, and pepper. Mix well until fully combined. • Press the mixture into the prepared loaf pan, smoothing the top with a spatula. • Bake for 45 minutes, or until firm and golden brown. • Allow to cool slightly before slicing and serving. **NUTRITIONAL FACTS (per Serving):** Calories: 350 | Total Fat: 8g | Saturated Fat: 1g | Fiber: 15g | Protein: 15g | Carbohydrate: 55g of which sugars: 7g | Vitamin A: 60% DV | Vitamin C: 15% DV | Calcium: 10% DV | Iron: 25% DV

STUFFED PORTOBELLO MUSHROOMS

Hearty and savory, these stuffed portobello mushrooms are filled with a delicious mixture of vegetables and herbs.

INGREDIENTS:	PREP TIME: 15 min	COOK TIME: 30 min	SERVINGS: 2 Servings

INGREDIENTS	INSTRUCTIONS:
4 large portobello mushrooms, stems removed 1 small onion, diced 1 red bell pepper, diced 1 zucchini, diced 2 cloves garlic, minced 1/4 cup breadcrumbs 1/4 cup grated vegan cheese (optional) 2 Tbsp olive oil 1 Tbsp fresh parsley, chopped 1 tsp dried thyme Salt and pepper to taste	• Preheat oven to 375°F (190°C). Line a baking sheet with parchment paper. • Brush portobello mushrooms with 1 Tbsp olive oil and place on the baking sheet. • In a skillet, heat remaining olive oil over medium heat. Add onion, red bell pepper, zucchini, and garlic. Sauté until vegetables are tender, about 5 minutes. • Stir in breadcrumbs, vegan cheese (if using), fresh parsley, dried thyme, salt, and pepper. • Fill each mushroom cap with the vegetable mixture. • Bake for 20-25 minutes, until mushrooms are tender and the filling is golden. • Serve warm. **NUTRITIONAL FACTS (per Serving):** Calories: 250 | Total Fat: 14g | Saturated Fat: 2g | Fiber: 6g | Protein: 7g | Carbohydrate: 28g of which sugars: 6g | Vitamin A: 30% DV | Vitamin C: 120% DV | Calcium: 8% DV | Iron: 10% DV

SPAGHETTI WITH WALNUT PESTO

A rich and nutty twist on classic pesto pasta, this dish is both delicious and easy to prepare.

INGREDIENTS:	PREP TIME: 10 min	COOK TIME: 10 min	SERVINGS: 2 Servings

INGREDIENTS:	INSTRUCTIONS:
4 oz spaghetti 1/2 cup walnuts, toasted 1 cup fresh basil leaves 1/4 cup grated Parmesan cheese (optional) 2 cloves garlic 1/4 cup olive oil 1 Tbsp lemon juice Salt and pepper to taste	• Cook spaghetti according to package instructions. Drain and set aside. • In a food processor, combine walnuts, basil leaves, Parmesan cheese (if using), garlic, olive oil, lemon juice, salt, and pepper. Process until smooth. • Toss the cooked spaghetti with the walnut pesto until well coated. • Serve immediately, garnished with additional Parmesan cheese and basil leaves if desired.
	NUTRITIONAL FACTS (per Serving): Calories: 450	Total Fat: 28g	Saturated Fat: 4.5g	Fiber: 4g	Protein: 12g	Carbohydrate: 40g of which sugars: 2g	Vitamin A: 20% DV	Vitamin C: 10% DV	Calcium: 15% DV	Iron: 15% DV

GRILLED VEGETABLE KEBABS WITH QUINOA

These colorful and nutritious vegetable kebabs are perfect when paired with fluffy quinoa for a complete meal.

INGREDIENTS:	PREP TIME: 15 min	COOK TIME: 20 min	SERVINGS: 2 Servings

INGREDIENTS:	INSTRUCTIONS:
1 red bell pepper, cut into chunks 1 yellow bell pepper, cut into chunks 1 zucchini, sliced 1 red onion, cut into chunks 8 cherry tomatoes 2 Tbsp olive oil 1 tsp dried oregano 1 tsp dried basil Salt and pepper to taste 1 cup quinoa, cooked	• Preheat grill to medium-high heat. • In a large bowl, toss the vegetables with olive oil, dried oregano, dried basil, salt, and pepper. • Thread the vegetables onto skewers. • Grill the kebabs for 15-20 minutes, turning occasionally, until the vegetables are tender and slightly charred. • Serve the grilled vegetable kebabs over a bed of cooked quinoa.
	NUTRITIONAL FACTS (per Serving): Calories: 350	Total Fat: 14g	Saturated Fat: 2g	Fiber: 8g	Protein: 10g	Carbohydrate: 50g of which sugars: 8g	Vitamin A: 70% DV	Vitamin C: 220% DV	Calcium: 6% DV	Iron: 20% DV

6. DESSERTS

RAW CASHEW CHEESECAKE

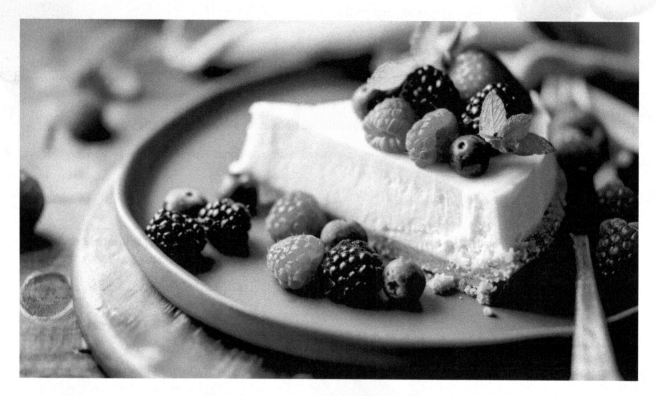

A creamy and delicious raw cashew cheesecake that's perfect for a healthy dessert.

INGREDIENTS:	PREP TIME: 10 min	COOK TIME: 0 min	SERVINGS: 2 Servings
1/2 cup almonds 1/2 cup dates, pitted 1 cup cashews, soaked for 4 hours 1/4 cup coconut oil, melted 1/4 cup maple syrup 1/4 cup lemon juice 1 tsp vanilla extract 1/2 cup mixed berries	**INSTRUCTIONS:** • In a food processor, blend almonds and dates until they form a sticky dough. Press the mixture into the bottom of a small springform pan to form the crust. • In a blender, combine soaked cashews, coconut oil, maple syrup, lemon juice, and vanilla extract. Blend until smooth and creamy. • Pour the filling over the crust and smooth the top with a spatula. • Freeze for at least 4 hours or until set. • Before serving, top with mixed berries.		
	NUTRITIONAL FACTS (per Serving): Calories: 380 | Total Fat: 28g | Saturated Fat: 12g | Fiber: 5g | Protein: 8g | Carbohydrate: 28g of which sugars: 16g | Vitamin A: 0% DV | Vitamin C: 15% DV | Calcium: 4% DV | Iron: 15% DV		

RAW CHOCOLATE AVOCADO MOUSSE

A creamy and indulgent dessert that combines the richness of avocado with the decadence of chocolate.

INGREDIENTS:	PREP TIME: 10 min	COOK TIME: 0 min	SERVINGS: 2 Servings

1 large ripe avocado 1/4 cup raw cocoa powder 1/4 cup maple syrup 1 tsp vanilla extract 1 pinch sea salt Fresh berries for garnish (optional)	**INSTRUCTIONS:** • Scoop the avocado flesh into a blender or food processor. • Add cocoa powder, maple syrup, vanilla extract, and sea salt. Blend until smooth and creamy. • Spoon the mousse into serving bowls and refrigerate for at least 30 minutes. • Garnish with fresh berries if desired before serving.
	NUTRITIONAL FACTS (per Serving): Calories: 250 | Total Fat: 15g | Saturated Fat: 2g | Fiber: 9g | Protein: 3g | Carbohydrate: 30g of which sugars: 20g | Vitamin A: 4% DV | Vitamin C: 20% DV | Calcium: 4% DV | Iron: 15% DV

BLUEBERRY AND CHIA SEED PUDDING

A refreshing and nutritious dessert made with chia seeds and fresh blueberries.

INGREDIENTS:	PREP TIME: 5 min	COOK TIME: 0 min	SERVINGS: 2 Servings

1 cup almond milk 1/4 cup chia seeds 1 Tbsp maple syrup 1/2 tsp vanilla extract 1/2 cup fresh blueberries	**INSTRUCTIONS:** • In a bowl, whisk together almond milk, chia seeds, maple syrup, and vanilla extract. • Let the mixture sit for 10 minutes, then whisk again to prevent clumping. • Cover and refrigerate for at least 2 hours or overnight until it thickens. • Divide the pudding into serving bowls and top with fresh blueberries before serving.
	NUTRITIONAL FACTS (per Serving): Calories: 180 | Total Fat: 8g | Saturated Fat: 0.5g | Fiber: 10g | Protein: 4g | Carbohydrate: 24g of which sugars: 10g | Vitamin A: 2% DV | Vitamin C: 15% DV | Calcium: 25% DV | Iron: 10% DV

VEGAN BANANA BREAD

A moist and flavorful vegan banana bread that's perfect for a healthy dessert or snack.

INGREDIENTS:	PREP TIME: 10 min	COOK TIME: 60 min	SERVINGS: 2 Servings
3 ripe bananas, mashed 1/4 cup maple syrup 1/4 cup coconut oil, melted 1 tsp vanilla extract 1 1/2 cups whole wheat flour 1 tsp baking soda 1/2 tsp ground cinnamon 1/4 tsp salt 1/2 cup walnuts, chopped (optional)	**INSTRUCTIONS:** • Preheat oven to 350°F (175°C). Grease a loaf pan. • In a large bowl, mix mashed bananas, maple syrup, coconut oil, and vanilla extract. • In a separate bowl, combine whole wheat flour, baking soda, ground cinnamon, and salt. • Add dry ingredients to wet ingredients and mix until just combined. Fold in walnuts if using. • Pour the batter into the prepared loaf pan and bake for 60 minutes or until a toothpick inserted into the center comes out clean. • Allow to cool before slicing and serving.		

NUTRITIONAL FACTS (per Serving): Calories: 320 | Total Fat: 14g | Saturated Fat: 6g | Fiber: 5g | Protein: 5g | Carbohydrate: 45g of which sugars: 15g | Vitamin A: 2% DV | Vitamin C: 6% DV | Calcium: 4% DV | Iron: 8% DV

COCONUT MILK ICE CREAM WITH BERRIES

A creamy and dairy-free ice cream made with coconut milk and topped with fresh berries.

INGREDIENTS:	PREP TIME: 10 min	COOK TIME: 0 min	SERVINGS: 2 Servings
1 can (14 oz) full-fat coconut milk 1/4 cup maple syrup 1 tsp vanilla extract 1 cup fresh berries (strawberries, blueberries, raspberries)	**INSTRUCTIONS:** • In a blender, combine coconut milk, maple syrup, and vanilla extract. Blend until smooth. • Pour the mixture into an ice cream maker and churn according to the manufacturer's instructions. • Once churned, transfer the ice cream to a container and freeze for at least 2 hours. • Serve topped with fresh berries.		

NUTRITIONAL FACTS (per Serving): Calories: 280 | Total Fat: 22g | Saturated Fat: 18g | Fiber: 3g | Protein: 2g | Carbohydrate: 22g of which sugars: 15g | Vitamin A: 0% DV | Vitamin C: 25% DV | Calcium: 2% DV | Iron: 10% DV

ALMOND FLOUR BROWNIES

These rich and fudgy almond flour brownies are a delicious and healthy treat.

INGREDIENTS:	PREP TIME: 10 min	COOK TIME: 25 min	SERVINGS: 2 Servings
1 cup almond flour 1/4 cup cocoa powder 1/4 tsp salt 1/4 tsp baking soda 1/2 cup maple syrup 1/4 cup coconut oil, melted 1 tsp vanilla extract 1/4 cup dark chocolate chips (optional)	**INSTRUCTIONS:** • Preheat oven to 350°F (175°C). Line a small baking pan with parchment paper. • In a bowl, mix almond flour, cocoa powder, salt, and baking soda. • In another bowl, combine maple syrup, melted coconut oil, and vanilla extract. • Add wet ingredients to dry ingredients and mix until combined. Fold in dark chocolate chips if using. • Pour the batter into the prepared pan and bake for 20-25 minutes until a toothpick inserted into the center comes out clean. • Let cool before cutting into squares and serving.		
	NUTRITIONAL FACTS (per Serving): Calories: 320 | Total Fat: 24g | Saturated Fat: 8g | Fiber: 6g | Protein: 6g | Carbohydrate: 28g of which sugars: 20g | Vitamin A: 0% DV | Vitamin C: 0% DV | Calcium: 6% DV | Iron: 10% DV		

MANGO COCONUT SORBET

A refreshing and tropical dessert, this mango coconut sorbet is perfect for a light and healthy treat.

INGREDIENTS:	PREP TIME: 10 min	COOK TIME: 0 min	SERVINGS: 2 Servings
2 ripe mangoes, peeled and chopped 1/2 cup coconut milk 2 Tbsp maple syrup 1 Tbsp lime juice	**INSTRUCTIONS:** • In a blender, combine chopped mangoes, coconut milk, maple syrup, and lime juice. Blend until smooth. • Pour the mixture into a freezer-safe container and freeze for at least 4 hours, stirring every 30 minutes to prevent ice crystals. • Scoop into bowls and serve.		
	NUTRITIONAL FACTS (per Serving): Calories: 150 | Total Fat: 7g | Saturated Fat: 6g | Fiber: 3g | Protein: 1g | Carbohydrate: 25g of which sugars: 22g | Vitamin A: 60% DV | Vitamin C: 80% DV | Calcium: 2% DV | Iron: 6% DV		

APPLE AND CINNAMON CRUMBLE

A warm and comforting dessert, this apple and cinnamon crumble is perfect for a cozy evening.

INGREDIENTS:	PREP TIME: 15 min	COOK TIME: 30 min	SERVINGS: 2 Servings
2 apples, peeled, cored, and sliced 1 Tbsp maple syrup 1 tsp ground cinnamon 1/2 tsp vanilla extract 1/2 cup rolled oats 1/4 cup almond flour 2 Tbsp coconut oil, melted 2 Tbsp maple syrup 1/4 tsp salt	**INSTRUCTIONS:** • Preheat oven to 350°F (175°C). Grease a small baking dish. • In a bowl, combine apple slices, maple syrup, ground cinnamon, and vanilla extract. Transfer to the baking dish. • In another bowl, mix rolled oats, almond flour, melted coconut oil, maple syrup, and salt until crumbly. • Sprinkle the crumble topping evenly over the apples. • Bake for 30 minutes until the topping is golden brown and the apples are tender. • Serve warm.		
	NUTRITIONAL FACTS (per Serving): Calories: 280 | Total Fat: 12g | Saturated Fat: 6g | Fiber: 5g | Protein: 3g | Carbohydrate: 42g of which sugars: 20g | Vitamin A: 2% DV | Vitamin C: 8% DV | Calcium: 4% DV | Iron: 6% DV		

BAKED PEARS WITH MAPLE SYRUP

A simple yet elegant dessert, baked pears with maple syrup offer a delightful and healthy sweet treat.

INGREDIENTS:	PREP TIME: 10 min	COOK TIME: 30 min	SERVINGS: 2 Servings
2 ripe pears, halved and cored 2 Tbsp maple syrup 1 tsp ground cinnamon 1/4 tsp ground nutmeg 1/4 cup chopped walnuts (optional) Fresh mint for garnish (optional)	**INSTRUCTIONS:** • Preheat oven to 375°F (190°C). Place pear halves in a baking dish, cut side up. • Drizzle pears with maple syrup and sprinkle with ground cinnamon and nutmeg. • Scatter chopped walnuts over the pears if using. • Bake for 25-30 minutes until pears are tender. • Garnish with fresh mint if desired and serve warm.		
	NUTRITIONAL FACTS (per Serving): Calories: 220 | Total Fat: 5g | Saturated Fat: 0.5g | Fiber: 6g | Protein: 2g | Carbohydrate: 45g of which sugars: 28g | Vitamin A: 2% DV | Vitamin C: 10% DV | Calcium: 4% DV | Iron: 4% DV		

MATCHA GREEN TEA COOKIES

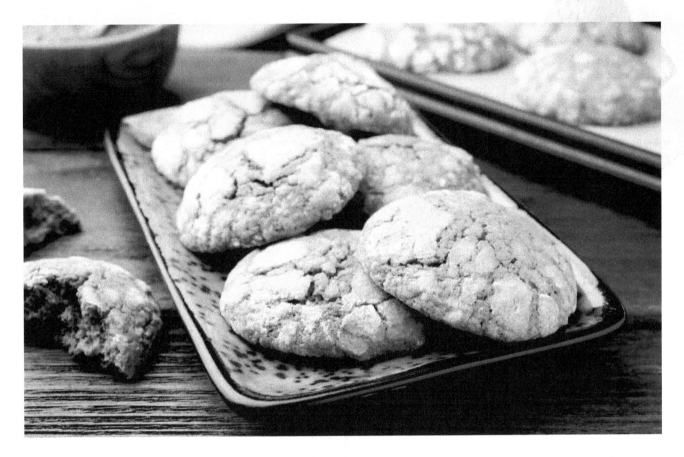

These vibrant and flavorful matcha green tea cookies are a delightful treat with a hint of earthy sweetness.

INGREDIENTS:	PREP TIME: 10 min	COOK TIME: 12 min	SERVINGS: 2 Servings
1 cup almond flour 2 Tbsp coconut flour 1 Tbsp matcha green tea powder 1/4 cup maple syrup 1/4 cup coconut oil, melted 1/2 tsp vanilla extract 1/4 tsp baking soda 1/8 tsp salt	**INSTRUCTIONS:** • Preheat oven to 350°F (175°C). Line a baking sheet with parchment paper. • In a bowl, mix almond flour, coconut flour, matcha powder, baking soda, and salt. • In another bowl, combine maple syrup, melted coconut oil, and vanilla extract. • Add wet ingredients to dry ingredients and mix until a dough forms. • Scoop tablespoons of dough onto the prepared baking sheet and flatten slightly. • Bake for 10-12 minutes until edges are golden. • Let cool before serving.		
	NUTRITIONAL FACTS (per Serving): Calories: 200 | Total Fat: 16g | Saturated Fat: 9g | Fiber: 3g | Protein: 4g | Carbohydrate: 14g of which sugars: 8g | Vitamin A: 0% DV | Vitamin C: 0% DV | Calcium: 6% DV | Iron: 6% DV		

DARK CHOCOLATE AND NUT CLUSTERS

A rich and satisfying dessert, these dark chocolate and nut clusters are easy to make and full of healthy fats.

INGREDIENTS:	PREP TIME: 10 min	COOK TIME: 0 min	SERVINGS: 2 Servings
1/2 cup dark chocolate chips (70% cacao or higher) 1/4 cup mixed nuts (almonds, walnuts, cashews) 1 Tbsp coconut oil 1/2 tsp vanilla extract 1 pinch sea salt	**INSTRUCTIONS:** • In a microwave-safe bowl, melt dark chocolate chips and coconut oil in 30-second intervals, stirring until smooth. • Stir in vanilla extract and mixed nuts until well coated. • Drop spoonfuls of the chocolate-nut mixture onto a parchment-lined baking sheet. • Sprinkle with sea salt. • Refrigerate for at least 1 hour until set. • Serve chilled.		
	NUTRITIONAL FACTS (per Serving): Calories: 240 | Total Fat: 18g | Saturated Fat: 8g | Fiber: 5g | Protein: 4g | Carbohydrate: 20g of which sugars: 12g | Vitamin A: 0% DV | Vitamin C: 0% DV | Calcium: 4% DV | Iron: 10% DV		

LEMON AND COCONUT ENERGY BALLS

These zesty and coconutty energy balls are perfect for a quick and healthy dessert or snack.

INGREDIENTS:	PREP TIME: 10 min	COOK TIME: 0 min	SERVINGS: 2 Servings
1/2 cup rolled oats 1/2 cup shredded coconut 1/4 cup almond flour 2 Tbsp maple syrup 1 Tbsp lemon juice 1 tsp lemon zest 1/4 tsp vanilla extract	**INSTRUCTIONS:** • In a food processor, combine rolled oats, shredded coconut, and almond flour. Pulse until finely ground. • Add maple syrup, lemon juice, lemon zest, and vanilla extract. Process until the mixture comes together. • Roll the mixture into small balls and place them on a parchment-lined baking sheet. • Chill in the refrigerator for at least 1 hour before serving.		
	NUTRITIONAL FACTS (per Serving): Calories: 200 | Total Fat: 10g | Saturated Fat: 6g | Fiber: 4g | Protein: 4g | Carbohydrate: 24g of which sugars: 10g | Vitamin A: 0% DV | Vitamin C: 8% DV | Calcium: 4% DV | Iron: 6% DV		

RAW VEGAN CARROT CAKE

A delicious and healthy raw vegan carrot cake that's perfect for a guilt-free dessert.

INGREDIENTS:	PREP TIME: 20 min	COOK TIME: 0 min	SERVINGS: 2 Servings
1 cup grated carrots 1/2 cup medjool dates, pitted 1/2 cup walnuts 1/4 cup shredded coconut 1/4 cup almond flour 1 tsp ground cinnamon 1/4 tsp ground nutmeg 1/4 tsp ground ginger 1/4 tsp salt 1/2 cup cashews, soaked for 4 hours 2 Tbsp coconut oil, melted 2 Tbsp maple syrup 1 Tbsp lemon juice 1/2 tsp vanilla extract 1-2 Tbsp water (as needed)	**INSTRUCTIONS:** • In a food processor, blend walnuts, shredded coconut, and almond flour until finely ground. Add grated carrots, dates, ground cinnamon, ground nutmeg, ground ginger, and salt. Process until the mixture sticks together. • Press the mixture into a small cake pan or form into a cake shape on a plate. • For the frosting, blend soaked cashews, melted coconut oil, maple syrup, lemon juice, and vanilla extract in a blender until smooth. Add water if needed to achieve a creamy consistency. • Spread the frosting over the cake and chill in the refrigerator for at least 2 hours before serving. **NUTRITIONAL FACTS (per Serving):** Calories: 380 | Total Fat: 26g | Saturated Fat: 10g | Fiber: 7g | Protein: 6g | Carbohydrate: 34g of which sugars: 20g | Vitamin A: 100% DV | Vitamin C: 8% DV | Calcium: 6% DV | Iron: 15% DV		

STRAWBERRY BASIL SORBET

A refreshing and unique sorbet that combines the sweetness of strawberries with the subtle flavor of basil.

INGREDIENTS:	PREP TIME: 10 min	COOK TIME: 0 min	SERVINGS: 2 Servings
2 cups fresh strawberries, hulled 1/4 cup fresh basil leaves 1/4 cup maple syrup 1 Tbsp lemon juice	**INSTRUCTIONS:** • In a blender, combine strawberries, basil leaves, maple syrup, and lemon juice. Blend until smooth. • Pour the mixture into a freezer-safe container and freeze for at least 4 hours, stirring every 30 minutes to prevent ice crystals. • Scoop into bowls and serve. **NUTRITIONAL FACTS (per Serving):** Calories: 100 | Total Fat: 0.5g | Saturated Fat: 0g | Fiber: 3g | Protein: 1g | Carbohydrate: 25g of which sugars: 20g | Vitamin A: 0% DV | Vitamin C: 90% DV | Calcium: 2% DV | Iron: 4% DV		

PUMPKIN SPICE COOKIES

These soft and flavorful pumpkin spice cookies are perfect for a healthy and comforting dessert.

INGREDIENTS:	PREP TIME: 10 min	COOK TIME: 15 min	SERVINGS: 2 Servings

INGREDIENTS	INSTRUCTIONS
1/2 cup pumpkin puree 1/4 cup maple syrup 2 Tbsp coconut oil, melted 1 tsp vanilla extract 1 cup almond flour 1/2 cup rolled oats 1 tsp ground cinnamon 1/2 tsp ground nutmeg 1/2 tsp ground ginger 1/4 tsp ground cloves 1/4 tsp baking soda 1/4 tsp salt	**INSTRUCTIONS:** • Preheat oven to 350°F (175°C). Line a baking sheet with parchment paper. • In a large bowl, combine pumpkin puree, maple syrup, melted coconut oil, and vanilla extract. • In a separate bowl, mix almond flour, rolled oats, ground cinnamon, ground nutmeg, ground ginger, ground cloves, baking soda, and salt. • Add dry ingredients to wet ingredients and mix until well combined. • Drop spoonfuls of dough onto the prepared baking sheet, flattening them slightly with the back of a spoon. • Bake for 12-15 minutes, until the cookies are golden brown. • Let cool before serving.

NUTRITIONAL FACTS (per Serving): Calories: 250 | Total Fat: 14g | Saturated Fat: 6g | Fiber: 5g | Protein: 6g | Carbohydrate: 28g of which sugars: 10g | Vitamin A: 60% DV | Vitamin C: 2% DV | Calcium: 6% DV | Iron: 10% DV

COCONUT MACAROONS

These chewy and sweet coconut macaroons are a delightful and simple dessert.

INGREDIENTS:	PREP TIME: 10 min	COOK TIME: 15 min	SERVINGS: 2 Servings

INGREDIENTS	INSTRUCTIONS
1 1/2 cups shredded coconut 1/4 cup almond flour 1/4 cup maple syrup 2 Tbsp coconut oil, melted 1 tsp vanilla extract 1/8 tsp salt	**INSTRUCTIONS:** • Preheat oven to 350°F (175°C). Line a baking sheet with parchment paper. • In a bowl, combine shredded coconut, almond flour, maple syrup, melted coconut oil, vanilla extract, and salt. • Mix until well combined and sticky. • Scoop tablespoons of the mixture onto the prepared baking sheet. • Bake for 12-15 minutes until golden brown. • Let cool before serving.

NUTRITIONAL FACTS (per Serving): Calories: 220 | Total Fat: 18g | Saturated Fat: 14g | Fiber: 5g | Protein: 3g | Carbohydrate: 16g of which sugars: 12g | Vitamin A: 0% DV | Vitamin C: 0% DV | Calcium: 2% DV | Iron: 4% DV

PINEAPPLE AND MINT PARFAIT

A refreshing and light dessert, this pineapple and mint parfait is perfect for a tropical twist.

INGREDIENTS:	PREP TIME: 10 min	COOK TIME: 0 min	SERVINGS: 2 Servings
1 cup fresh pineapple, diced 1 cup coconut yogurt 2 Tbsp shredded coconut 1 Tbsp fresh mint, chopped 1 Tbsp maple syrup (optional)	**INSTRUCTIONS:** • In a bowl, mix the coconut yogurt with maple syrup if using. • In serving glasses, layer the pineapple, coconut yogurt, and shredded coconut. • Garnish with fresh mint. • Serve immediately.		
	NUTRITIONAL FACTS (per Serving): Calories: 160 | Total Fat: 7g | Saturated Fat: 6g | Fiber: 3g | Protein: 2g | Carbohydrate: 22g of which sugars: 15g | Vitamin A: 2% DV | Vitamin C: 70% DV | Calcium: 2% DV | Iron: 4% DV		

CHOCOLATE-DIPPED STRAWBERRIES

A classic and elegant dessert, these chocolate-dipped strawberries are both simple and delightful.

INGREDIENTS:	PREP TIME: 10 min	COOK TIME: 0 min	SERVINGS: 2 Servings
1 cup fresh strawberries 1/2 cup dark chocolate chips (70% cacao or higher) 1 Tbsp coconut oil	**INSTRUCTIONS:** • Wash and dry the strawberries, leaving the stems intact. • In a microwave-safe bowl, melt dark chocolate chips and coconut oil in 30-second intervals, stirring until smooth. • Dip each strawberry into the melted chocolate, allowing the excess to drip off. • Place the dipped strawberries on a parchment-lined baking sheet. • Refrigerate for at least 30 minutes until the chocolate is set. • Serve chilled.		
	NUTRITIONAL FACTS (per Serving): Calories: 200 | Total Fat: 14g | Saturated Fat: 9g | Fiber: 5g | Protein: 2g | Carbohydrate: 20g of which sugars: 14g | Vitamin A: 0% DV | Vitamin C: 80% DV | Calcium: 2% DV | Iron: 10% DV		

RAW LEMON BARS

These tangy and sweet raw lemon bars are a refreshing and healthy dessert option.

INGREDIENTS:	PREP TIME: 15 min	COOK TIME: 0 min	SERVINGS: 2 Servings
1/2 cup almonds 1/2 cup dates, pitted 1/4 cup shredded coconut 1 cup cashews, soaked for 4 hours 1/4 cup coconut oil, melted 1/4 cup maple syrup 1/4 cup lemon juice 1 tsp lemon zest	**INSTRUCTIONS:** • In a food processor, blend almonds, dates, and shredded coconut until it forms a sticky dough. Press the mixture into the bottom of a small baking dish. • In a blender, combine soaked cashews, melted coconut oil, maple syrup, lemon juice, and lemon zest. Blend until smooth and creamy. • Pour the filling over the crust and smooth the top with a spatula. • Freeze for at least 2 hours until set. • Cut into bars and serve chilled.		
	NUTRITIONAL FACTS (per Serving): Calories: 300 | Total Fat: 22g | Saturated Fat: 10g | Fiber: 4g | Protein: 6g | Carbohydrate: 25g of which sugars: 16g | Vitamin A: 0% DV | Vitamin C: 15% DV | Calcium: 4% DV | Iron: 10% DV		

CHIA SEED AND RASPBERRY JAM

A simple and healthy homemade jam made with chia seeds and fresh raspberries.

INGREDIENTS:	PREP TIME: 5 min	COOK TIME: 5 min	SERVINGS: 2 Servings
1 cup fresh raspberries 1 Tbsp chia seeds 1 Tbsp maple syrup 1 tsp lemon juice	**INSTRUCTIONS:** • In a small saucepan, cook raspberries over medium heat until they start to break down, about 5 minutes. • Remove from heat and stir in chia seeds, maple syrup, and lemon juice. • Let the mixture sit for 10 minutes to thicken. • Transfer to a jar and refrigerate for at least 1 hour before serving.		
	NUTRITIONAL FACTS (per Serving): Calories: 80 | Total Fat: 2.5g | Saturated Fat: 0g | Fiber: 8g | Protein: 1g | Carbohydrate: 15g of which sugars: 10g | Vitamin A: 0% DV | Vitamin C: 30% DV | Calcium: 4% DV | Iron: 4% DV		

7. SMOOTHIES AND BEVERAGES

BERRY AND BEET SMOOTHIE

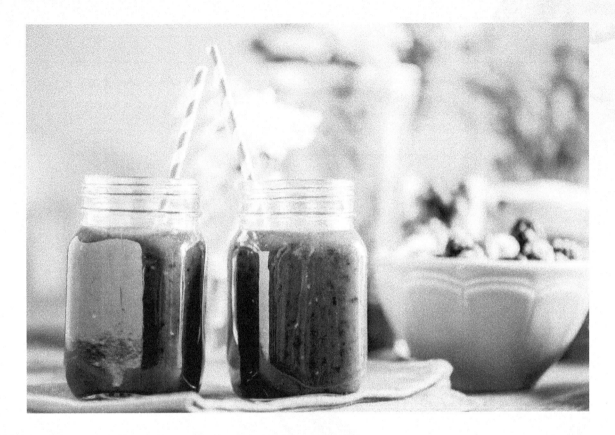

A delicious and nutrient-packed smoothie with the sweetness of berries and the earthy richness of beets.

INGREDIENTS:	PREP TIME: 5 min	COOK TIME: 0 min	SERVINGS: 2 Servings
1 small beet, peeled and chopped 1/2 cup strawberries 1/2 cup blueberries 1/2 banana 1 cup almond milk 1 Tbsp flaxseeds 1 tsp honey (optional)	**INSTRUCTIONS:** • In a blender, combine beet, strawberries, blueberries, banana, almond milk, flaxseeds, and honey if using. • Blend until smooth. • Pour into glasses and serve immediately.		
	NUTRITIONAL FACTS (per Serving): Calories: 200 | Total Fat: 5g | Saturated Fat: 0.5g | Fiber: 8g | Protein: 4g | Carbohydrate: 38g of which sugars: 20g | Vitamin A: 2% DV | Vitamin C: 60% DV | Calcium: 25% DV | Iron: 10% DV		

GREEN DETOX SMOOTHIE

This vibrant and refreshing green detox smoothie is perfect for a nutritious start to your day.

INGREDIENTS:	PREP TIME: 5 min	COOK TIME: 0 min	SERVINGS: 2 Servings
1 cup spinach 1/2 cucumber, chopped 1 green apple, cored and chopped 1/2 avocado 1 Tbsp fresh lemon juice 1 cup coconut water 1 Tbsp chia seeds 1 tsp fresh ginger, grated	**INSTRUCTIONS:** • In a blender, combine spinach, cucumber, green apple, avocado, lemon juice, coconut water, chia seeds, and fresh ginger. • Blend until smooth and creamy. • Pour into glasses and serve immediately.		
	NUTRITIONAL FACTS (per Serving): Calories: 180 | Total Fat: 9g | Saturated Fat: 1.5g | Fiber: 10g | Protein: 3g | Carbohydrate: 24g of which sugars: 10g | Vitamin A: 50% DV | Vitamin C: 40% DV | Calcium: 8% DV | Iron: 15% DV		

TROPICAL MANGO AND PINEAPPLE SMOOTHIE

This tropical smoothie combines the sweetness of mango and pineapple for a refreshing and nutritious beverage.

INGREDIENTS:	PREP TIME: 5 min	COOK TIME: 0 min	SERVINGS: 2 Servings
1 cup frozen mango chunks 1 cup frozen pineapple chunks 1 banana 1 cup coconut water 1 Tbsp chia seeds 1 tsp fresh lime juice	**INSTRUCTIONS:** • In a blender, combine mango, pineapple, banana, coconut water, chia seeds, and lime juice. • Blend until smooth and creamy. • Pour into glasses and serve immediately.		
	NUTRITIONAL FACTS (per Serving): Calories: 210 | Total Fat: 3g | Saturated Fat: 1g | Fiber: 7g | Protein: 3g | Carbohydrate: 50g of which sugars: 35g | Vitamin A: 50% DV | Vitamin C: 150% DV | Calcium: 4% DV | Iron: 6% DV		

ALMOND AND DATE SMOOTHIE

A rich and creamy smoothie with the natural sweetness of dates and the nutty flavor of almonds.

INGREDIENTS:	PREP TIME: 5 min	COOK TIME: 0 min	SERVINGS: 2 Servings

INGREDIENTS:	INSTRUCTIONS:
1 cup almond milk 4 dates, pitted 1/4 cup almonds 1 banana 1 Tbsp almond butter 1/2 tsp vanilla extract	• In a blender, combine almond milk, dates, almonds, banana, almond butter, and vanilla extract. • Blend until smooth and creamy. • Pour into glasses and serve immediately.

NUTRITIONAL FACTS (per Serving): Calories: 280 | Total Fat: 12g | Saturated Fat: 1g | Fiber: 6g | Protein: 6g | Carbohydrate: 42g of which sugars: 28g | Vitamin A: 2% DV | Vitamin C: 10% DV | Calcium: 20% DV | Iron: 8% DV

SPINACH AND BANANA SMOOTHIE

This creamy and nutritious smoothie combines the benefits of spinach with the sweetness of banana for a delicious and healthy drink.

INGREDIENTS:	PREP TIME: 5 min	COOK TIME: 0 min	SERVINGS: 2 Servings

INGREDIENTS:	INSTRUCTIONS:
2 cups fresh spinach 1 banana 1 cup almond milk 1 Tbsp almond butter 1 tsp honey (optional) 1/2 tsp vanilla extract	• In a blender, combine spinach, banana, almond milk, almond butter, honey (if using), and vanilla extract. • Blend until smooth and creamy. • Pour into glasses and serve immediately.

NUTRITIONAL FACTS (per Serving): Calories: 180 | Total Fat: 8g | Saturated Fat: 1g | Fiber: 4g | Protein: 4g | Carbohydrate: 24g of which sugars: 14g | Vitamin A: 80% DV | Vitamin C: 30% DV | Calcium: 25% DV | Iron: 8% DV

MATCHA GREEN TEA LATTE

A soothing and energizing matcha green tea latte, perfect for a healthy beverage any time of day.

INGREDIENTS:	PREP TIME: 5 min	COOK TIME: 5 min	SERVINGS: 2 Servings
2 tsp matcha green tea powder 1 cup almond milk 1 cup water 1 Tbsp maple syrup (optional) 1/2 tsp vanilla extract	**INSTRUCTIONS:** • In a small bowl, whisk the matcha green tea powder with a few tablespoons of hot water to make a smooth paste. • In a saucepan, heat the almond milk and remaining water over medium heat until warm but not boiling. • Whisk in the matcha paste, maple syrup (if using), and vanilla extract until well combined. • Pour into mugs and serve warm.		
	NUTRITIONAL FACTS (per Serving): Calories: 60	Total Fat: 2g	Saturated Fat: 0.5g	Fiber: 1g	Protein: 1g	Carbohydrate: 8g of which sugars: 4g	Vitamin A: 2% DV	Vitamin C: 0% DV	Calcium: 20% DV	Iron: 4% DV		

TURMERIC GOLDEN MILK

A warming and soothing drink, turmeric golden milk is perfect for an anti-inflammatory boost.

INGREDIENTS:	PREP TIME: 5 min	COOK TIME: 5 min	SERVINGS: 2 Servings
2 cups almond milk 1 tsp ground turmeric 1/2 tsp ground cinnamon 1/2 tsp ground ginger 1 Tbsp maple syrup 1/2 tsp vanilla extract 1 pinch black pepper	**INSTRUCTIONS:** • In a small saucepan, combine almond milk, ground turmeric, ground cinnamon, ground ginger, maple syrup, vanilla extract, and black pepper. • Heat over medium heat, stirring frequently, until warm but not boiling. • Pour into mugs and serve warm.		
	NUTRITIONAL FACTS (per Serving): Calories: 90	Total Fat: 3g	Saturated Fat: 0.5g	Fiber: 2g	Protein: 1g	Carbohydrate: 14g of which sugars: 10g	Vitamin A: 0% DV	Vitamin C: 0% DV	Calcium: 25% DV	Iron: 6% DV		

CARROT AND GINGER JUICE

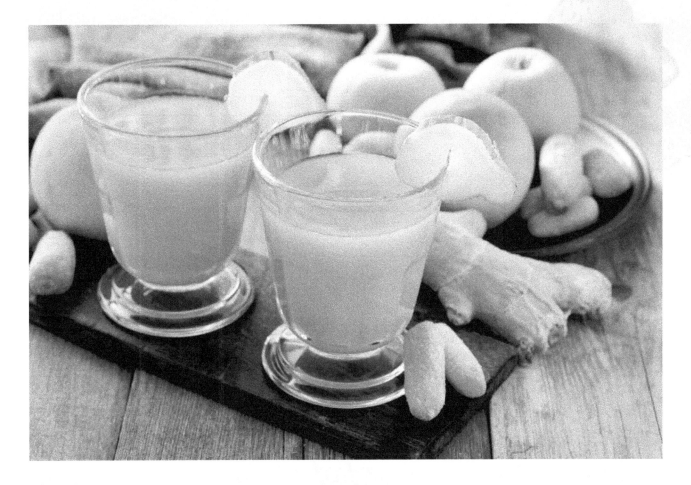

A vibrant and healthy juice that combines the sweetness of carrots with the zing of ginger.

INGREDIENTS:	PREP TIME: 5 min	COOK TIME: 0 min	SERVINGS: 2 Servings

INGREDIENTS:

4 large carrots, peeled and chopped

1-inch piece fresh ginger, peeled and chopped

1 apple, cored and chopped

1 cup water

1 Tbsp fresh lemon juice

INSTRUCTIONS:

- In a blender, combine carrots, ginger, apple, water, and lemon juice.

- Blend until smooth.

- Strain the juice to remove pulp if desired.

- Pour into glasses and serve immediately.

NUTRITIONAL FACTS (per Serving): Calories: 90 | Total Fat: 0.5g | Saturated Fat: 0g | Fiber: 4g | Protein: 1g | Carbohydrate: 22g of which sugars: 15g | Vitamin A: 400% DV | Vitamin C: 20% DV | Calcium: 4% DV | Iron: 2% DV

WATERMELON MINT COOLER

This refreshing and hydrating cooler is perfect for hot days, combining the sweetness of watermelon with the freshness of mint.

INGREDIENTS:	PREP TIME: 5 min	COOK TIME: 0 min	SERVINGS: 2 Servings

INGREDIENTS:	INSTRUCTIONS:
3 cups watermelon, cubed 1 Tbsp fresh lime juice 1/4 cup fresh mint leaves 1 cup cold water Ice cubes	• In a blender, combine watermelon, lime juice, mint leaves, and cold water. • Blend until smooth. • Pour into glasses over ice cubes and serve immediately.

NUTRITIONAL FACTS (per Serving): Calories: 50 | Total Fat: 0g | Saturated Fat: 0g | Fiber: 1g | Protein: 1g | Carbohydrate: 12g of which sugars: 9g | Vitamin A: 15% DV | Vitamin C: 25% DV | Calcium: 2% DV | Iron: 2% DV

CHIA FRESCA

A hydrating and energizing drink, chia fresca is perfect for a natural boost of energy and hydration.

INGREDIENTS:	PREP TIME: 5 min	COOK TIME: 0 min	SERVINGS: 2 Servings

INGREDIENTS:	INSTRUCTIONS:
2 cups water 2 Tbsp chia seeds 1 Tbsp fresh lemon juice 1 Tbsp honey or maple syrup 1/4 tsp vanilla extract (optional)	• In a large glass or jar, combine water, chia seeds, lemon juice, honey or maple syrup, and vanilla extract if using. • Stir well to combine and let sit for 10-15 minutes, stirring occasionally, until the chia seeds swell and form a gel-like consistency. • Stir again before serving and enjoy chilled.

NUTRITIONAL FACTS (per Serving): Calories: 70 | Total Fat: 3g | Saturated Fat: 0g | Fiber: 6g | Protein: 2g | Carbohydrate: 9g of which sugars: 6g | Vitamin A: 0% DV | Vitamin C: 10% DV | Calcium: 8% DV | Iron: 6% DV

SPICED APPLE CIDER

This warm and comforting spiced apple cider is perfect for cozy evenings and holiday gatherings.

INGREDIENTS:	PREP TIME: 5 min	COOK TIME: 20 min	SERVINGS: 2 Servings
2 cups apple cider 1 cinnamon stick 2 whole cloves 1 star anise 1 orange slice 1 Tbsp maple syrup 1 tsp fresh ginger, grated	**INSTRUCTIONS:** • In a saucepan, combine apple cider, cinnamon stick, cloves, star anise, orange slice, maple syrup, and grated ginger. • Bring to a simmer over medium heat and cook for 20 minutes. • Strain the cider to remove the spices and orange slice. • Pour into mugs and serve warm.		
	NUTRITIONAL FACTS (per Serving): Calories: 120 | Total Fat: 0g | Saturated Fat: 0g | Fiber: 1g | Protein: 0g | Carbohydrate: 30g of which sugars: 28g | Vitamin A: 2% DV | Vitamin C: 8% DV | Calcium: 4% DV | Iron: 2% DV		

COCONUT WATER AND BERRY SMOOTHIE

A light and refreshing smoothie, this coconut water and berry blend is perfect for hydration and a burst of antioxidants.

INGREDIENTS:	PREP TIME: 5 min	COOK TIME: 0 min	SERVINGS: 2 Servings
1 cup coconut water 1/2 cup strawberries 1/2 cup blueberries 1/2 banana 1 Tbsp chia seeds 1 tsp honey (optional)	**INSTRUCTIONS:** • In a blender, combine coconut water, strawberries, blueberries, banana, chia seeds, and honey if using. • Blend until smooth and creamy. • Pour into glasses and serve immediately.		
	NUTRITIONAL FACTS (per Serving): Calories: 120 | Total Fat: 2g | Saturated Fat: 0g | Fiber: 5g | Protein: 2g | Carbohydrate: 26g of which sugars: 16g | Vitamin A: 0% DV | Vitamin C: 60% DV | Calcium: 4% DV | Iron: 4% DV		

POMEGRANATE AND ORANGE JUICE

A vibrant and refreshing juice that combines the sweetness of oranges with the tanginess of pomegranates.

INGREDIENTS:	PREP TIME: 5 min	COOK TIME: 0 min	SERVINGS: 2 Servings

INGREDIENTS	INSTRUCTIONS
1 cup pomegranate seeds 2 large oranges, juiced 1 Tbsp lemon juice 1 tsp honey (optional) Ice cubes	**INSTRUCTIONS:** • In a blender, combine pomegranate seeds, orange juice, lemon juice, and honey if using. • Blend until smooth. • Strain the juice to remove the pulp if desired. • Pour into glasses over ice cubes and serve immediately.

NUTRITIONAL FACTS (per Serving): Calories: 120 | Total Fat: 0.5g | Saturated Fat: 0g | Fiber: 4g | Protein: 2g | Carbohydrate: 30g of which sugars: 26g | Vitamin A: 6% DV | Vitamin C: 90% DV | Calcium: 4% DV | Iron: 2% DV

HERBAL DETOX TEA

A soothing and cleansing herbal detox tea to help flush out toxins and support overall health.

INGREDIENTS:	PREP TIME: 5 min	COOK TIME: 10 min	SERVINGS: 2 Servings

INGREDIENTS	INSTRUCTIONS
2 cups water 1 tsp dried dandelion root 1 tsp dried burdock root 1 tsp dried nettle leaves 1 tsp fresh ginger, grated 1 Tbsp fresh lemon juice 1 tsp honey (optional)	**INSTRUCTIONS:** • In a small saucepan, bring water to a boil. • Add dandelion root, burdock root, nettle leaves, and grated ginger. • Reduce heat and let it simmer for 10 minutes. • Strain the tea into cups, then add lemon juice and honey if using. • Serve warm.

NUTRITIONAL FACTS (per Serving): Calories: 15 | Total Fat: 0g | Saturated Fat: 0g | Fiber: 0g | Protein: 0g | Carbohydrate: 4g of which sugars: 2g | Vitamin A: 0% DV | Vitamin C: 10% DV | Calcium: 4% DV | Iron: 2% DV

CUCUMBER AND ALOE VERA JUICE

A hydrating and soothing juice, perfect for cooling down on a hot day.

INGREDIENTS:	PREP TIME: 5 min	COOK TIME: 0 min	SERVINGS: 2 Servings

1 large cucumber, peeled and chopped 2 Tbsp fresh aloe vera gel 1 cup water 1 Tbsp fresh lime juice 1 tsp honey (optional)	**INSTRUCTIONS:** • In a blender, combine cucumber, aloe vera gel, water, lime juice, and honey if using. • Blend until smooth. • Strain the juice to remove any pulp if desired. • Pour into glasses and serve immediately.
	NUTRITIONAL FACTS (per Serving): Calories: 40	Total Fat: 0g	Saturated Fat: 0g	Fiber: 1g	Protein: 1g	Carbohydrate: 10g of which sugars: 5g	Vitamin A: 2% DV	Vitamin C: 15% DV	Calcium: 2% DV	Iron: 2% DV

PINEAPPLE AND TURMERIC SMOOTHIE

This vibrant and anti-inflammatory smoothie combines the sweetness of pineapple with the powerful benefits of turmeric.

INGREDIENTS:	PREP TIME: 5 min	COOK TIME: 0 min	SERVINGS: 2 Servings

1 cup pineapple chunks (fresh or frozen) 1 banana 1 cup coconut water 1/2 tsp ground turmeric 1/4 tsp ground ginger 1 Tbsp chia seeds 1 tsp honey (optional)	**INSTRUCTIONS:** • In a blender, combine pineapple chunks, banana, coconut water, ground turmeric, ground ginger, chia seeds, and honey if using. • Blend until smooth and creamy. • Pour into glasses and serve immediately.
	NUTRITIONAL FACTS (per Serving): Calories: 150	Total Fat: 2g	Saturated Fat: 0.5g	Fiber: 5g	Protein: 2g	Carbohydrate: 34g of which sugars: 22g	Vitamin A: 2% DV	Vitamin C: 70% DV	Calcium: 6% DV	Iron: 6% DV

ICED HIBISCUS TEA

This refreshing and tart iced hibiscus tea is perfect for cooling down on a hot day and is packed with antioxidants.

INGREDIENTS:	PREP TIME: 5 min	COOK TIME: 10 min	SERVINGS: 2 Servings

INGREDIENTS:	INSTRUCTIONS:
2 cups water 2 Tbsp dried hibiscus flowers 1 Tbsp fresh lime juice 1 Tbsp honey or maple syrup (optional) Ice cubes Fresh mint leaves for garnish (optional)	• In a small saucepan, bring water to a boil. Remove from heat and add dried hibiscus flowers. • Let steep for 10 minutes. • Strain the tea into a pitcher and stir in lime juice and honey or maple syrup if using. • Refrigerate until chilled. • Serve over ice and garnish with fresh mint leaves if desired.

NUTRITIONAL FACTS (per Serving): Calories: 30 | Total Fat: 0g | Saturated Fat: 0g | Fiber: 0g | Protein: 0g | Carbohydrate: 8g of which sugars: 6g | Vitamin A: 0% DV | Vitamin C: 15% DV | Calcium: 2% DV | Iron: 2% DV

GINGER AND LEMON INFUSED WATER

A refreshing and detoxifying drink, perfect for hydration and boosting your immune system.

INGREDIENTS:	PREP TIME: 5 min	COOK TIME: 0 min	SERVINGS: 2 Servings

INGREDIENTS:	INSTRUCTIONS:
4 cups water 1-inch piece fresh ginger, sliced 1 lemon, sliced Fresh mint leaves (optional)	• In a large pitcher, combine water, sliced ginger, and sliced lemon. • Add fresh mint leaves if using. • Refrigerate for at least 1 hour to allow the flavors to infuse. • Serve chilled.

NUTRITIONAL FACTS (per Serving): Calories: 5 | Total Fat: 0g | Saturated Fat: 0g | Fiber: 0g | Protein: 0g | Carbohydrate: 1g of which sugars: 0g | Vitamin A: 0% DV | Vitamin C: 10% DV | Calcium: 0% DV | Iron: 0% DV

8. SALADS AND SIDES

SPINACH AND STRAWBERRY SALAD

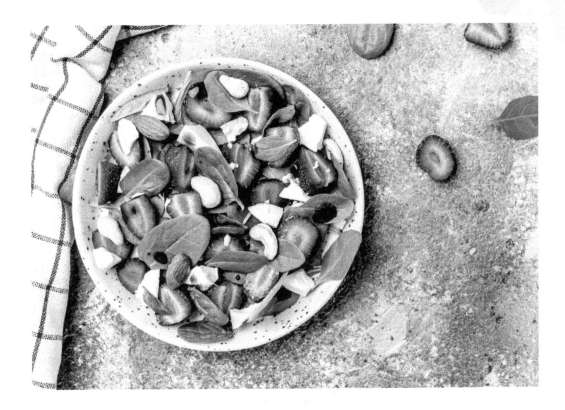

A refreshing and vibrant salad combining the sweetness of strawberries with the earthiness of spinach.

INGREDIENTS:	PREP TIME: 10 min	COOK TIME: 0 min	SERVINGS: 2 Servings
2 cups fresh spinach leaves 1 cup strawberries, sliced 1/4 red onion, thinly sliced 1/4 cup crumbled feta cheese 1/4 cup sliced almonds, toasted 2 Tbsp balsamic vinaigrette	**INSTRUCTIONS:** • In a large bowl, combine spinach, strawberries, red onion, feta cheese, and sliced almonds. • Drizzle with balsamic vinaigrette and toss gently to combine. • Serve immediately.		
	NUTRITIONAL FACTS (per Serving): Calories: 190 | Total Fat: 12g | Saturated Fat: 3g | Fiber: 4g | Protein: 6g | Carbohydrate: 16g of which sugars: 8g | Vitamin A: 50% DV | Vitamin C: 90% DV | Calcium: 15% DV | Iron: 10% DV		

ROASTED BRUSSELS SPROUTS WITH BALSAMIC GLAZE

A delicious side dish featuring crispy roasted Brussels sprouts with a tangy balsamic glaze.

INGREDIENTS:	PREP TIME: 10 min	COOK TIME: 25 min	SERVINGS: 2 Servings

INGREDIENTS	INSTRUCTIONS
2 cups Brussels sprouts, trimmed and halved 1 Tbsp olive oil 1/2 tsp sea salt 1/4 tsp black pepper 2 Tbsp balsamic vinegar 1 Tbsp maple syrup	**INSTRUCTIONS:** • Preheat the oven to 400°F (200°C). • Toss Brussels sprouts with olive oil, sea salt, and black pepper. • Spread on a baking sheet and roast for 20-25 minutes until crispy and golden. • In a small saucepan, heat balsamic vinegar and maple syrup over medium heat until reduced by half. • Drizzle the balsamic glaze over the roasted Brussels sprouts before serving.

NUTRITIONAL FACTS (per Serving): Calories: 150 | Total Fat: 7g | Saturated Fat: 1g | Fiber: 5g | Protein: 4g | Carbohydrate: 20g of which sugars: 10g | Vitamin A: 15% DV | Vitamin C: 120% DV | Calcium: 6% DV | Iron: 10% DV

BEET AND ARUGULA SALAD WITH GOAT CHEESE

A vibrant and nutritious salad combining the earthy flavors of beets with the peppery bite of arugula and creamy goat cheese.

INGREDIENTS:	PREP TIME: 10 min	COOK TIME: 40 min	SERVINGS: 2 Servings

INGREDIENTS	INSTRUCTIONS
2 medium beets, roasted and sliced 2 cups arugula 1/4 cup crumbled goat cheese 1/4 cup walnuts, toasted 1 Tbsp olive oil 1 Tbsp balsamic vinegar 1 tsp honey Salt and pepper to taste	**INSTRUCTIONS:** • Preheat the oven to 400°F (200°C). Wrap beets in foil and roast for 35-40 minutes until tender. Let cool, then slice. • In a large bowl, combine arugula, roasted beets, goat cheese, and toasted walnuts. • In a small bowl, whisk together olive oil, balsamic vinegar, honey, salt, and pepper. • Drizzle the dressing over the salad and toss to combine.

NUTRITIONAL FACTS (per Serving): Calories: 250 | Total Fat: 15g | Saturated Fat: 4g | Fiber: 5g | Protein: 7g | Carbohydrate: 22g of which sugars: 14g | Vitamin A: 15% DV | Vitamin C: 20% DV | Calcium: 8% DV | Iron: 10% DV

CUCUMBER AND TOMATO SALAD WITH DILL

A light and refreshing salad featuring crisp cucumbers, juicy tomatoes, and aromatic dill.

INGREDIENTS:	PREP TIME: 10 min	COOK TIME: 0 min	SERVINGS: 2 Servings
1 cucumber, sliced 1 cup cherry tomatoes, halved 1/4 red onion, thinly sliced 2 Tbsp fresh dill, chopped 1 Tbsp olive oil 1 Tbsp apple cider vinegar Salt and pepper to taste	**INSTRUCTIONS:** • In a large bowl, combine cucumber, cherry tomatoes, red onion, and fresh dill. • In a small bowl, whisk together olive oil, apple cider vinegar, salt, and pepper. • Pour the dressing over the salad and toss to combine. • Serve immediately or refrigerate for 30 minutes to allow flavors to meld.		
	NUTRITIONAL FACTS (per Serving): Calories: 70 | Total Fat: 5g | Saturated Fat: 0.5g | Fiber: 2g | Protein: 1g | Carbohydrate: 7g of which sugars: 4g | Vitamin A: 10% DV | Vitamin C: 25% DV | Calcium: 2% DV | Iron: 2% DV		

SWEET POTATO FRIES WITH AVOCADO DIP

Crispy and healthy sweet potato fries served with a creamy avocado dip for a perfect side dish.

INGREDIENTS:	PREP TIME: 10 min	COOK TIME: 25 min	SERVINGS: 2 Servings
2 medium sweet potatoes, cut into fries 1 Tbsp olive oil 1/2 tsp paprika 1/2 tsp garlic powder 1/4 tsp sea salt 1 ripe avocado 2 Tbsp Greek yogurt 1 Tbsp fresh lime juice 1 Tbsp fresh cilantro, chopped Salt and pepper to taste	**INSTRUCTIONS:** • Preheat the oven to 425°F (220°C). • Toss sweet potato fries with olive oil, paprika, garlic powder, and sea salt. Spread on a baking sheet in a single layer. • Bake for 20-25 minutes until crispy, turning halfway through. • In a small bowl, mash the avocado and mix with Greek yogurt, lime juice, cilantro, salt, and pepper. • Serve the sweet potato fries with avocado dip.		
	NUTRITIONAL FACTS (per Serving): Calories: 250 | Total Fat: 14g | Saturated Fat: 2g | Fiber: 8g | Protein: 4g | Carbohydrate: 30g of which sugars: 8g | Vitamin A: 400% DV | Vitamin C: 35% DV | Calcium: 4% DV | Iron: 6% DV		

GRILLED ASPARAGUS WITH LEMON ZEST

A simple and flavorful side dish, grilled asparagus with a hint of lemon zest.

INGREDIENTS:	PREP TIME: 5 min	COOK TIME: 10 min	SERVINGS: 2 Servings

INGREDIENTS	INSTRUCTIONS
1 bunch asparagus, trimmed 1 Tbsp olive oil 1 tsp lemon zest Salt and pepper to taste Lemon wedges for serving	**INSTRUCTIONS:** • Preheat the grill to medium-high heat. • Toss asparagus with olive oil, salt, and pepper. • Grill asparagus for 5-7 minutes, turning occasionally until tender and slightly charred. • Remove from grill and sprinkle with lemon zest. • Serve with lemon wedges.

NUTRITIONAL FACTS (per Serving): Calories: 70 | Total Fat: 5g | Saturated Fat: 0.5g | Fiber: 3g | Protein: 2g | Carbohydrate: 6g of which sugars: 2g | Vitamin A: 20% DV | Vitamin C: 30% DV | Calcium: 4% DV | Iron: 15% DV

BROCCOLI AND RAISIN SALAD

A sweet and savory salad featuring crunchy broccoli and sweet raisins, perfect for a nutritious side dish.

INGREDIENTS:	PREP TIME: 10 min	COOK TIME: 0 min	SERVINGS: 2 Servings

INGREDIENTS	INSTRUCTIONS
2 cups broccoli florets 1/4 cup raisins 1/4 cup red onion, finely chopped 2 Tbsp sunflower seeds 2 Tbsp Greek yogurt 1 Tbsp apple cider vinegar 1 tsp honey Salt and pepper to taste	**INSTRUCTIONS:** • In a large bowl, combine broccoli florets, raisins, red onion, and sunflower seeds. • In a small bowl, whisk together Greek yogurt, apple cider vinegar, honey, salt, and pepper. • Pour the dressing over the broccoli mixture and toss to combine. • Serve immediately or chill for an hour to let the flavors meld.

NUTRITIONAL FACTS (per Serving): Calories: 150 | Total Fat: 6g | Saturated Fat: 0.5g | Fiber: 4g | Protein: 4g | Carbohydrate: 22g of which sugars: 12g | Vitamin A: 15% DV | Vitamin C: 120% DV | Calcium: 8% DV | Iron: 8% DV

ROASTED CARROT AND FENNEL SALAD

A beautifully roasted carrot and fennel salad, perfect as a side dish with its sweet and savory flavors.

INGREDIENTS:	PREP TIME: 10 min	COOK TIME: 25 min	SERVINGS: 2 Servings
4 large carrots, peeled and cut into sticks 1 bulb fennel, sliced 1 Tbsp olive oil 1 tsp fresh thyme, chopped 1 Tbsp balsamic vinegar Salt and pepper to taste 2 Tbsp pumpkin seeds (optional)	**INSTRUCTIONS:** • Preheat the oven to 400°F (200°C). • Toss carrots and fennel with olive oil, thyme, salt, and pepper. Spread on a baking sheet. • Roast for 20-25 minutes, until tender and caramelized. • Drizzle with balsamic vinegar and sprinkle with pumpkin seeds if using. • Serve warm or at room temperature.		
	NUTRITIONAL FACTS (per Serving): Calories: 150 | Total Fat: 7g | Saturated Fat: 1g | Fiber: 6g | Protein: 2g | Carbohydrate: 20g of which sugars: 10g | Vitamin A: 350% DV | Vitamin C: 20% DV | Calcium: 6% DV | Iron: 6% DV		

SPICED CAULIFLOWER BITES

These spiced cauliflower bites are a tasty and healthy alternative to traditional fried snacks, perfect as a side or appetizer.

INGREDIENTS:	PREP TIME: 10 min	COOK TIME: 25 min	SERVINGS: 2 Servings
1 medium cauliflower, cut into florets 2 Tbsp olive oil 1 tsp smoked paprika 1/2 tsp ground cumin 1/2 tsp garlic powder 1/4 tsp cayenne pepper Salt and pepper to taste Fresh parsley for garnish (optional)	**INSTRUCTIONS:** • Preheat the oven to 400°F (200°C). • In a large bowl, toss cauliflower florets with olive oil, smoked paprika, cumin, garlic powder, cayenne pepper, salt, and pepper. • Spread the cauliflower on a baking sheet in a single layer. • Roast for 20-25 minutes, until tender and slightly crispy. • Garnish with fresh parsley if desired and serve warm.		
	NUTRITIONAL FACTS (per Serving): Calories: 180 | Total Fat: 14g | Saturated Fat: 2g | Fiber: 5g | Protein: 3g | Carbohydrate: 12g of which sugars: 3g | Vitamin A: 10% DV | Vitamin C: 90% DV | Calcium: 4% DV | Iron: 6% DV		

ZESTY COLESLAW WITH APPLE

A tangy and refreshing coleslaw with a hint of sweetness from fresh apples, perfect for a light side dish.

INGREDIENTS:	PREP TIME: 10 min	COOK TIME: 0 min	SERVINGS: 2 Servings
2 cups shredded cabbage 1 carrot, grated 1 apple, julienned 1/4 cup Greek yogurt 1 Tbsp apple cider vinegar 1 tsp honey 1/2 tsp Dijon mustard Salt and pepper to taste	**INSTRUCTIONS:** • In a large bowl, combine shredded cabbage, grated carrot, and julienned apple. • In a small bowl, whisk together Greek yogurt, apple cider vinegar, honey, Dijon mustard, salt, and pepper. • Pour the dressing over the cabbage mixture and toss to coat. • Serve immediately or refrigerate for 30 minutes to let the flavors meld.		
	NUTRITIONAL FACTS (per Serving): Calories: 100 | Total Fat: 1g | Saturated Fat: 0.5g | Fiber: 4g | Protein: 3g | Carbohydrate: 20g of which sugars: 12g | Vitamin A: 60% DV | Vitamin C: 70% DV | Calcium: 6% DV | Iron: 4% DV		

GARLIC AND HERB ROASTED POTATOES

Crispy on the outside and tender on the inside, these garlic and herb roasted potatoes are a perfect side for any meal.

INGREDIENTS:	PREP TIME: 10 min	COOK TIME: 30 min	SERVINGS: 2 Servings
4 small potatoes, quartered 2 Tbsp olive oil 2 cloves garlic, minced 1 tsp dried rosemary 1 tsp dried thyme Salt and pepper to taste Fresh parsley, chopped (for garnish)	**INSTRUCTIONS:** • Preheat the oven to 425°F (220°C). • In a large bowl, toss quartered potatoes with olive oil, minced garlic, dried rosemary, dried thyme, salt, and pepper. • Spread the potatoes on a baking sheet in a single layer. • Roast for 25-30 minutes, until golden and crispy, turning halfway through. • Garnish with fresh parsley and serve warm.		
	NUTRITIONAL FACTS (per Serving): Calories: 220 | Total Fat: 14g | Saturated Fat: 2g | Fiber: 4g | Protein: 3g | Carbohydrate: 22g of which sugars: 2g | Vitamin A: 2% DV | Vitamin C: 25% DV | Calcium: 4% DV | Iron: 6% DV		

AVOCADO AND CORN SALAD

A refreshing and creamy salad featuring the smooth texture of avocado with the sweet crunch of corn.

INGREDIENTS:	PREP TIME: 10 min	COOK TIME: 0 min	SERVINGS: 2 Servings
1 avocado, diced 1 cup corn kernels (fresh or thawed if frozen) 1/2 red bell pepper, diced 1/4 red onion, finely chopped 2 Tbsp fresh cilantro, chopped 1 Tbsp fresh lime juice 1 Tbsp olive oil Salt and pepper to taste	**INSTRUCTIONS:** • In a large bowl, combine diced avocado, corn kernels, red bell pepper, red onion, and fresh cilantro. • In a small bowl, whisk together lime juice, olive oil, salt, and pepper. • Pour the dressing over the salad and toss gently to combine. • Serve immediately.		
	NUTRITIONAL FACTS (per Serving): Calories: 200 | Total Fat: 15g | Saturated Fat: 2g | Fiber: 6g | Protein: 3g | Carbohydrate: 18g of which sugars: 5g | Vitamin A: 15% DV | Vitamin C: 60% DV | Calcium: 2% DV | Iron: 6% DV		

MARINATED MUSHROOM SALAD

A savory and tangy salad with marinated mushrooms, perfect as a flavorful side dish.

INGREDIENTS:	PREP TIME: 10 min	COOK TIME: 0 min	SERVINGS: 2 Servings
2 cups button mushrooms, sliced 1/4 cup red onion, thinly sliced 1/4 cup olive oil 2 Tbsp red wine vinegar 1 clove garlic, minced 1 tsp Dijon mustard 1 tsp fresh thyme, chopped Salt and pepper to taste	**INSTRUCTIONS:** • In a large bowl, combine sliced mushrooms and red onion. • In a small bowl, whisk together olive oil, red wine vinegar, minced garlic, Dijon mustard, fresh thyme, salt, and pepper. • Pour the dressing over the mushroom mixture and toss to coat. • Cover and refrigerate for at least 1 hour to marinate. • Serve chilled or at room temperature.		
	NUTRITIONAL FACTS (per Serving): Calories: 180 | Total Fat: 16g | Saturated Fat: 2.5g | Fiber: 2g | Protein: 2g | Carbohydrate: 8g of which sugars: 4g | Vitamin A: 2% DV | Vitamin C: 10% DV | Calcium: 2% DV | Iron: 6% DV		

MIXED GREENS WITH CITRUS VINAIGRETTE

A light and refreshing salad with mixed greens and a tangy citrus vinaigrette.

INGREDIENTS:	PREP TIME: 10 min	COOK TIME: 0 min	SERVINGS: 2 Servings
4 cups mixed salad greens 1/2 cup cherry tomatoes, halved 1/4 red onion, thinly sliced 1/4 cup cucumber, sliced 2 Tbsp olive oil 2 Tbsp fresh orange juice 1 Tbsp fresh lemon juice 1 tsp Dijon mustard Salt and pepper to taste	**INSTRUCTIONS:** • In a large bowl, combine mixed salad greens, cherry tomatoes, red onion, and cucumber. • In a small bowl, whisk together olive oil, orange juice, lemon juice, Dijon mustard, salt, and pepper. • Drizzle the vinaigrette over the salad and toss to combine. • Serve immediately.		
	NUTRITIONAL FACTS (per Serving): Calories: 120 | Total Fat: 10g | Saturated Fat: 1.5g | Fiber: 3g | Protein: 2g | Carbohydrate: 9g of which sugars: 4g | Vitamin A: 60% DV | Vitamin C: 50% DV | Calcium: 6% DV | Iron: 8% DV		

ROASTED BEET AND ORANGE SALAD

A colorful and nutritious salad featuring roasted beets and fresh oranges, perfect for a refreshing side.

INGREDIENTS:	PREP TIME: 10 min	COOK TIME: 40 min	SERVINGS: 2 Servings
2 medium beets, roasted and sliced 1 orange, peeled and segmented 2 cups arugula 1/4 red onion, thinly sliced 1/4 cup crumbled goat cheese 2 Tbsp walnuts, toasted 2 Tbsp olive oil 1 Tbsp balsamic vinegar Salt and pepper to taste	**INSTRUCTIONS:** • Preheat the oven to 400°F (200°C). Wrap beets in foil and roast for 35-40 minutes until tender. Let cool, then slice. • In a large bowl, combine roasted beets, orange segments, arugula, red onion, goat cheese, and walnuts. • In a small bowl, whisk together olive oil, balsamic vinegar, salt, and pepper. • Drizzle the dressing over the salad and toss to combine. • Serve immediately.		
	NUTRITIONAL FACTS (per Serving): Calories: 250 | Total Fat: 14g | Saturated Fat: 3g | Fiber: 5g | Protein: 6g | Carbohydrate: 27g of which sugars: 16g | Vitamin A: 25% DV | Vitamin C: 50% DV | Calcium: 10% DV | Iron: 10% DV		

GRILLED ZUCCHINI WITH MINT

A refreshing and light side dish, grilled zucchini with a touch of fresh mint is perfect for any meal.

INGREDIENTS:	PREP TIME: 10 min	COOK TIME: 10 min	SERVINGS: 2 Servings
2 medium zucchinis, sliced lengthwise 1 Tbsp olive oil Salt and pepper to taste 2 Tbsp fresh mint leaves, chopped 1 Tbsp fresh lemon juice	**INSTRUCTIONS:** • Preheat the grill to medium-high heat. • Brush zucchini slices with olive oil and season with salt and pepper. • Grill zucchini for 3-4 minutes on each side, until tender and grill marks appear. • Remove from grill and drizzle with lemon juice. • Sprinkle with fresh mint leaves and serve warm.		
	NUTRITIONAL FACTS (per Serving): Calories: 100 | Total Fat: 7g | Saturated Fat: 1g | Fiber: 2g | Protein: 2g | Carbohydrate: 8g of which sugars: 4g | Vitamin A: 10% DV | Vitamin C: 30% DV | Calcium: 4% DV | Iron: 4% DV		

PARSNIP AND CARROT MASH

A creamy and flavorful mash, combining the earthy sweetness of parsnips and carrots.

INGREDIENTS:	PREP TIME: 10 min	COOK TIME: 20 min	SERVINGS: 2 Servings
2 large parsnips, peeled and chopped 2 large carrots, peeled and chopped 1 Tbsp olive oil 2 Tbsp Greek yogurt Salt and pepper to taste 1 Tbsp fresh parsley, chopped	**INSTRUCTIONS:** • In a large pot, bring water to a boil. Add parsnips and carrots, and cook until tender, about 15-20 minutes. • Drain and transfer to a bowl. • Mash the parsnips and carrots with olive oil and Greek yogurt until smooth. • Season with salt and pepper. • Garnish with fresh parsley and serve warm.		
	NUTRITIONAL FACTS (per Serving): Calories: 150 | Total Fat: 7g | Saturated Fat: 1g | Fiber: 6g | Protein: 2g | Carbohydrate: 22g of which sugars: 10g | Vitamin A: 240% DV | Vitamin C: 30% DV | Calcium: 8% DV | Iron: 4% DV		

9. SPECIAL DIETS

NUT-FREE ENERGY BARS

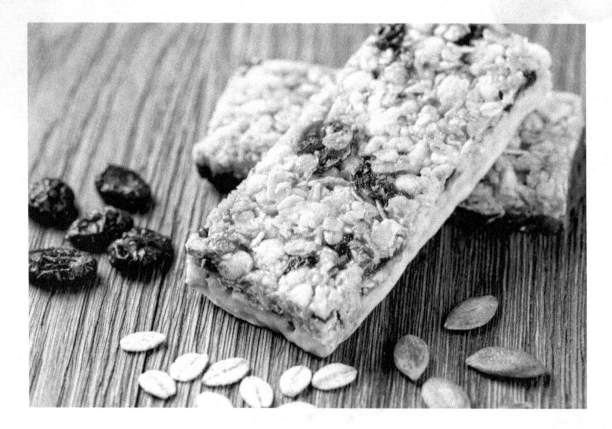

These nut-free energy bars are perfect for a quick and healthy snack on the go.

INGREDIENTS:	PREP TIME: 10 min	COOK TIME: 0 min	SERVINGS: 2 Servings
1 cup rolled oats 1/4 cup sunflower seeds 1/4 cup pumpkin seeds 1/4 cup dried cranberries 1/4 cup shredded coconut 2 Tbsp chia seeds 1/4 cup sunflower seed butter 1/4 cup honey or maple syrup 1/2 tsp vanilla extract	**INSTRUCTIONS:** • In a large bowl, combine oats, sunflower seeds, pumpkin seeds, dried cranberries, shredded coconut, and chia seeds. • In a small saucepan, heat sunflower seed butter, honey or maple syrup, and vanilla extract over low heat until smooth. • Pour the warm mixture over the dry ingredients and mix well. • Press the mixture into a lined baking dish and refrigerate for at least 2 hours until firm. • Cut into bars and serve.		
	NUTRITIONAL FACTS (per Serving): Calories: 250 | Total Fat: 12g | Saturated Fat: 3g | Fiber: 6g | Protein: 6g | Carbohydrate: 30g of which sugars: 15g | Vitamin A: 0% DV | Vitamin C: 2% DV | Calcium: 4% DV | Iron: 10% DV		

GLUTEN-FREE BUCKWHEAT PANCAKES

These fluffy and nutritious buckwheat pancakes are perfect for a gluten-free breakfast.

INGREDIENTS:	PREP TIME: 10 min	COOK TIME: 15 min	SERVINGS: 2 Servings
1 cup buckwheat flour 1 Tbsp ground flaxseed 1 Tbsp maple syrup 1 tsp baking powder 1/2 tsp baking soda 1/4 tsp salt 1 cup almond milk 1 tsp apple cider vinegar 1 Tbsp coconut oil (for cooking)	**INSTRUCTIONS:** • In a large bowl, whisk together buckwheat flour, ground flaxseed, baking powder, baking soda, and salt. • In a separate bowl, mix almond milk, apple cider vinegar, and maple syrup. Let sit for a few minutes to curdle. • Combine the wet and dry ingredients, stirring until just combined. • Heat a non-stick skillet over medium heat and add coconut oil. • Pour batter onto the skillet, cooking until bubbles form and edges are set, then flip and cook until golden brown. • Serve warm with your favorite toppings.		
	NUTRITIONAL FACTS (per Serving): Calories: 250 | Total Fat: 10g | Saturated Fat: 4g | Fiber: 5g | Protein: 6g | Carbohydrate: 35g of which sugars: 6g | Vitamin A: 0% DV | Vitamin C: 0% DV | Calcium: 20% DV | Iron: 10% DV		

DAIRY-FREE ALFREDO PASTA

A creamy and delicious dairy-free Alfredo pasta, perfect for those avoiding dairy.

INGREDIENTS:	PREP TIME: 10 min	COOK TIME: 15 min	SERVINGS: 2 Servings
8 oz gluten-free pasta 1 cup unsweetened almond milk 1/2 cup raw cashews, soaked and drained 2 Tbsp nutritional yeast 1 clove garlic, minced 1 Tbsp olive oil 1 Tbsp lemon juice Salt and pepper to taste Fresh parsley for garnish (optional)	**INSTRUCTIONS:** • Cook pasta according to package instructions, then drain and set aside. • In a blender, combine almond milk, soaked cashews, nutritional yeast, garlic, olive oil, lemon juice, salt, and pepper. Blend until smooth and creamy. • In a large skillet, heat the sauce over medium heat until warm. • Add the cooked pasta to the skillet and toss to coat with the sauce. • Serve immediately, garnished with fresh parsley if desired.		
	NUTRITIONAL FACTS (per Serving): Calories: 400 | Total Fat: 18g | Saturated Fat: 2.5g | Fiber: 5g | Protein: 12g | Carbohydrate: 54g of which sugars: 2g | Vitamin A: 2% DV | Vitamin C: 4% DV | Calcium: 15% DV | Iron: 20% DV		

LOW-SUGAR BERRY CRUMBLE

A delightful and healthy dessert, this low-sugar berry crumble is perfect for satisfying your sweet tooth without the guilt.

INGREDIENTS:	PREP TIME: 10 min	COOK TIME: 25 min	SERVINGS: 2 Servings
1 cup mixed berries (blueberries, raspberries, strawberries) 1 Tbsp fresh lemon juice 1 Tbsp chia seeds 1 Tbsp honey (optional) 1/2 cup rolled oats 1/4 cup almond flour 2 Tbsp coconut oil, melted 1/2 tsp cinnamon 1/4 tsp salt	**INSTRUCTIONS:** • Preheat the oven to 350°F (175°C). • In a bowl, mix berries, lemon juice, chia seeds, and honey if using. Spread the mixture in a small baking dish. • In another bowl, combine oats, almond flour, coconut oil, cinnamon, and salt. Mix until crumbly. • Sprinkle the oat mixture over the berries. • Bake for 20-25 minutes until the topping is golden and the berries are bubbly. • Let cool slightly before serving.		
	NUTRITIONAL FACTS (per Serving): Calories: 200	Total Fat: 10g	Saturated Fat: 6g	Fiber: 6g	Protein: 4g	Carbohydrate: 26g of which sugars: 2g	Vitamin A: 2% DV	Vitamin C: 35% DV	Calcium: 6% DV	Iron: 8% DV		

ANTI-INFLAMMATORY TURMERIC SOUP

This warming and nutritious turmeric soup is packed with anti-inflammatory ingredients to help soothe and heal your body.

INGREDIENTS:	PREP TIME: 10 min	COOK TIME: 25 min	SERVINGS: 2 Servings
1 Tbsp olive oil 1 onion, chopped 2 cloves garlic, minced 1 carrot, diced 1 celery stalk, diced 1 tsp ground turmeric 1/2 tsp ground ginger 4 cups vegetable broth 1 cup chopped kale 1/2 cup coconut milk Salt and pepper to taste Lemon wedges for serving	**INSTRUCTIONS:** • In a large pot, heat olive oil over medium heat. Sauté onion, garlic, carrot, and celery until softened, about 5 minutes. • Add turmeric and ginger, cooking for another minute. • Pour in vegetable broth and bring to a boil. Reduce heat and simmer for 15 minutes. • Stir in chopped kale and coconut milk, cooking for an additional 5 minutes. • Season with salt and pepper, and serve with lemon wedges.		
	NUTRITIONAL FACTS (per Serving): Calories: 150	Total Fat: 10g	Saturated Fat: 4g	Fiber: 3g	Protein: 4g	Carbohydrate: 14g of which sugars: 4g	Vitamin A: 110% DV	Vitamin C: 70% DV	Calcium: 10% DV	Iron: 15% DV		

PROTEIN-PACKED VEGAN CHILI

A hearty and nutritious vegan chili loaded with protein-rich ingredients, perfect for a satisfying meal.

INGREDIENTS:	PREP TIME: 15 min	COOK TIME: 30 min	SERVINGS: 2 Servings

INGREDIENTS	INSTRUCTIONS
1 Tbsp olive oil 1 onion, chopped 2 cloves garlic, minced 1 bell pepper, chopped 1 cup cooked quinoa 1 can (15 oz) black beans, drained and rinsed 1 can (15 oz) kidney beans, drained and rinsed 1 can (15 oz) diced tomatoes 1 cup vegetable broth 1 Tbsp chili powder 1 tsp ground cumin 1/2 tsp smoked paprika Salt and pepper to taste	**INSTRUCTIONS:** • In a large pot, heat olive oil over medium heat. Sauté onion, garlic, and bell pepper until softened, about 5 minutes. • Add cooked quinoa, black beans, kidney beans, diced tomatoes, and vegetable broth. Stir to combine. • Add chili powder, ground cumin, smoked paprika, salt, and pepper. • Bring to a boil, then reduce heat and simmer for 20 minutes, stirring occasionally. • Serve hot.

NUTRITIONAL FACTS (per Serving): Calories: 350 | Total Fat: 7g | Saturated Fat: 1g | Fiber: 15g | Protein: 18g | Carbohydrate: 55g of which sugars: 8g | Vitamin A: 25% DV | Vitamin C: 50% DV | Calcium: 15% DV | Iron: 35% DV

PALEO-STYLE CAULIFLOWER RICE BOWL

A healthy and satisfying paleo dish, this cauliflower rice bowl is loaded with vegetables and flavorful seasonings.

INGREDIENTS:	PREP TIME: 10 min	COOK TIME: 15 min	SERVINGS: 2 Servings

INGREDIENTS	INSTRUCTIONS
1 small head cauliflower, riced 1 Tbsp coconut oil 1 bell pepper, diced 1 zucchini, diced 1 cup spinach leaves 1/2 cup cherry tomatoes, halved 1/2 avocado, sliced 2 Tbsp coconut aminos 1 tsp sesame seeds Salt and pepper to taste	**INSTRUCTIONS:** • In a large skillet, heat coconut oil over medium heat. Add riced cauliflower and cook for 5 minutes. • Add bell pepper, zucchini, and spinach, sautéing until vegetables are tender, about 7-10 minutes. • Stir in cherry tomatoes and coconut aminos, cooking for another 2 minutes. • Season with salt and pepper. • Serve the cauliflower rice in bowls, topped with avocado slices and sesame seeds.

NUTRITIONAL FACTS (per Serving): Calories: 250 | Total Fat: 16g | Saturated Fat: 7g | Fiber: 8g | Protein: 5g | Carbohydrate: 24g of which sugars: 9g | Vitamin A: 70% DV | Vitamin C: 120% DV | Calcium: 6% DV | Iron: 10% DV

KETO-FRIENDLY AVOCADO SALAD

A delicious and satisfying keto-friendly salad featuring creamy avocado and fresh vegetables.

INGREDIENTS:	PREP TIME: 10 min	COOK TIME: 0 min	SERVINGS: 2 Servings

INGREDIENTS:	INSTRUCTIONS:
2 avocados, diced 1/2 cucumber, diced 1/2 red bell pepper, diced 1/4 red onion, finely chopped 1/4 cup fresh cilantro, chopped 2 Tbsp lime juice 1 Tbsp olive oil Salt and pepper to taste	• In a large bowl, combine diced avocado, cucumber, red bell pepper, red onion, and cilantro. • In a small bowl, whisk together lime juice, olive oil, salt, and pepper. • Pour the dressing over the salad and toss gently to combine. • Serve immediately

NUTRITIONAL FACTS (per Serving): Calories: 280 | Total Fat: 25g | Saturated Fat: 3.5g | Fiber: 10g | Protein: 3g | Carbohydrate: 15g of which sugars: 4g | Vitamin A: 15% DV | Vitamin C: 60% DV | Calcium: 2% DV | Iron: 6% DV

VEGAN LENTIL LOAF

A hearty and flavorful vegan lentil loaf, perfect for a wholesome dinner.

INGREDIENTS:	PREP TIME: 15 min	COOK TIME: 45 min	SERVINGS: 2 Servings

INGREDIENTS:	INSTRUCTIONS:
1 cup cooked lentils 1/2 cup rolled oats 1/4 cup finely chopped onion 1/4 cup grated carrot 2 Tbsp ground flaxseed mixed with 6 Tbsp water 2 Tbsp tomato paste 1 Tbsp soy sauce or tamari 1 tsp garlic powder 1 tsp dried thyme Salt and pepper to taste 1/4 cup ketchup (for topping)	• Preheat the oven to 375°F (190°C). Line a loaf pan with parchment paper. • In a large bowl, combine cooked lentils, rolled oats, onion, carrot, flaxseed mixture, tomato paste, soy sauce, garlic powder, dried thyme, salt, and pepper. Mix well. • Press the mixture into the prepared loaf pan. • Spread ketchup on top of the loaf. • Bake for 45 minutes until firm and golden brown. • Let cool slightly before slicing and serving.

NUTRITIONAL FACTS (per Serving): Calories: 320 | Total Fat: 7g | Saturated Fat: 1g | Fiber: 14g | Protein: 14g | Carbohydrate: 50g of which sugars: 10g | Vitamin A: 60% DV | Vitamin C: 15% DV | Calcium: 8% DV | Iron: 30% DV

10. HEALING AND DETOX

ALKALINE GREEN SOUP

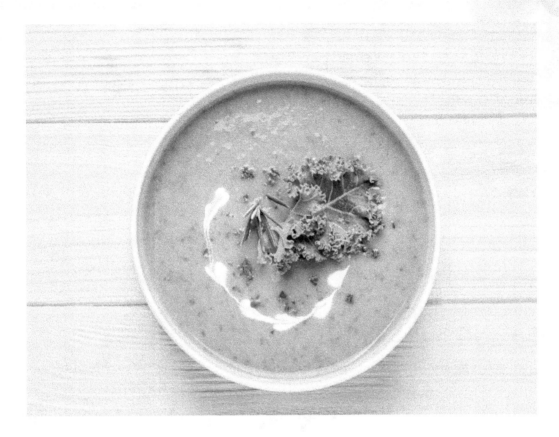

A nourishing and detoxifying soup, perfect for supporting your body's natural pH balance.

INGREDIENTS:	PREP TIME: 10 min	COOK TIME: 20 min	SERVINGS: 2 Servings
1 Tbsp olive oil 1 onion, chopped 2 cloves garlic, minced 1 zucchini, chopped 1 cup broccoli florets 2 cups spinach leaves 1 celery stalk, chopped 4 cups vegetable broth 1/2 lemon, juiced Salt and pepper to taste	**INSTRUCTIONS:** • In a large pot, heat olive oil over medium heat. Sauté onion and garlic until softened, about 5 minutes. • Add zucchini, broccoli, spinach, and celery, cooking for another 5 minutes. • Pour in vegetable broth and bring to a boil. Reduce heat and simmer for 10 minutes. • Blend the soup until smooth using an immersion blender or in batches in a blender. • Stir in lemon juice, season with salt and pepper, and serve warm.		
	NUTRITIONAL FACTS (per Serving): Calories: 120 | Total Fat: 7g | Saturated Fat: 1g | Fiber: 4g | Protein: 4g | Carbohydrate: 14g of which sugars: 6g | Vitamin A: 80% DV | Vitamin C: 150% DV | Calcium: 10% DV | Iron: 15% DV		

LIVER DETOX SMOOTHIE

A refreshing smoothie packed with liver-supporting ingredients to help detoxify and cleanse your body.

INGREDIENTS:	PREP TIME: 10 min	COOK TIME: 0 min	SERVINGS: 2 Servings

INGREDIENTS:	
1 cup kale leaves	**INSTRUCTIONS:**
1/2 cup cucumber, chopped	
1 green apple, chopped	• Add all ingredients to a blender.
1/2 lemon, juiced	• Blend until smooth.
1-inch piece of ginger, peeled	• Serve immediately.
1/4 cup fresh parsley	
1 cup coconut water	

NUTRITIONAL FACTS (per Serving): Calories: 90 | Total Fat: 0.5g | Saturated Fat: 0g | Fiber: 5g | Protein: 2g | Carbohydrate: 20g of which sugars: 10g | Vitamin A: 60% DV | Vitamin C: 90% DV | Calcium: 10% DV | Iron: 10% DV

GUT-HEALING BONE BROTH

A nourishing and soothing broth rich in collagen and amino acids to support gut health and overall well-being.

INGREDIENTS:	PREP TIME: 10 min	COOK TIME: 4-6 h	SERVINGS: 2 Servings

INGREDIENTS:	
2 lbs chicken bones (preferably organic)	**INSTRUCTIONS:**
1 onion, quartered	• Place all ingredients in a large pot or slow cooker.
2 carrots, chopped	• Bring to a boil, then reduce heat and simmer for 4-6 hours, skimming any foam that rises to the top.
2 celery stalks, chopped	
2 cloves garlic, smashed	• Strain the broth through a fine mesh sieve.
1 Tbsp apple cider vinegar	• Serve warm, garnished with fresh parsley if desired.
8 cups water	
1 tsp sea salt	
1 tsp black peppercorns	
2 bay leaves	
Fresh parsley for garnish (optional)	

NUTRITIONAL FACTS (per Serving): Calories: 150 | Total Fat: 5g | Saturated Fat: 1.5g | Fiber: 1g | Protein: 20g | Carbohydrate: 4g of which sugars: 2g | Vitamin A: 50% DV | Vitamin C: 10% DV | Calcium: 6% DV | Iron: 8% DV

ANTI-INFLAMMATORY GOLDEN MILK

A warm and soothing beverage rich in anti-inflammatory compounds to help reduce inflammation and promote overall health.

INGREDIENTS:	PREP TIME: 5 min	COOK TIME: 5 min	SERVINGS: 2 Servings

INGREDIENTS:	INSTRUCTIONS:
2 cups unsweetened almond milk 1 tsp ground turmeric 1/2 tsp ground cinnamon 1/4 tsp ground ginger 1 Tbsp coconut oil 1 Tbsp honey or maple syrup (optional) Pinch of black pepper	• In a small saucepan, heat almond milk over medium heat until warm. • Whisk in turmeric, cinnamon, ginger, coconut oil, honey or maple syrup, and black pepper until well combined. • Continue to heat for another 2-3 minutes, stirring frequently. • Pour into mugs and serve warm.

NUTRITIONAL FACTS (per Serving): Calories: 120 | Total Fat: 10g | Saturated Fat: 4g | Fiber: 2g | Protein: 2g | Carbohydrate: 8g of which sugars: 5g | Vitamin A: 2% DV | Vitamin C: 0% DV | Calcium: 25% DV | Iron: 10% DV

IMMUNE-BOOSTING GARLIC SOUP

A comforting and immune-boosting garlic soup, perfect for warding off colds and flu.

INGREDIENTS:	PREP TIME: 10 min	COOK TIME: 20 min	SERVINGS: 2 Servings

INGREDIENTS:	INSTRUCTIONS:
1 Tbsp olive oil 1 onion, chopped 1 head of garlic, peeled and minced 2 carrots, chopped 2 celery stalks, chopped 4 cups vegetable broth 1 tsp thyme 1 tsp rosemary Salt and pepper to taste Fresh parsley for garnish (optional)	• In a large pot, heat olive oil over medium heat. Sauté onion and garlic until fragrant, about 5 minutes. • Add carrots and celery, cooking for another 5 minutes. • Pour in vegetable broth and bring to a boil. Reduce heat and simmer for 10 minutes. • Add thyme, rosemary, salt, and pepper. • Serve warm, garnished with fresh parsley if desired.

NUTRITIONAL FACTS (per Serving): Calories: 150 | Total Fat: 6g | Saturated Fat: 1g | Fiber: 5g | Protein: 4g | Carbohydrate: 20g of which sugars: 8g | Vitamin A: 120% DV | Vitamin C: 15% DV | Calcium: 8% DV | Iron: 6% DV

CLEANSING BEET JUICE

A vibrant and nutrient-packed juice, perfect for detoxifying the body and boosting overall health.

INGREDIENTS:	PREP TIME: 10 min	COOK TIME: 0 min	SERVINGS: 2 Servings

INGREDIENTS:

2 medium beets, peeled and chopped

1 green apple, chopped

1 carrot, chopped

1/2 lemon, juiced

1-inch piece of ginger, peeled

1 cup water

INSTRUCTIONS:

- Add all ingredients to a blender.
- Blend until smooth.
- Strain through a fine mesh sieve or nut milk bag if desired.
- Serve immediately.

NUTRITIONAL FACTS (per Serving): Calories: 90 | Total Fat: 0.5g | Saturated Fat: 0g | Fiber: 5g | Protein: 2g | Carbohydrate: 20g of which sugars: 14g | Vitamin A: 60% DV | Vitamin C: 25% DV | Calcium: 4% DV | Iron: 6% DV

HEALING TURMERIC AND GINGER TEA

A soothing and healing tea with anti-inflammatory properties, perfect for boosting immunity and reducing inflammation.

INGREDIENTS:	PREP TIME: 5 min	COOK TIME: 10 min	SERVINGS: 2 Servings

INGREDIENTS:

2 cups water

1 tsp ground turmeric

1-inch piece of ginger, peeled and sliced

1 Tbsp honey or maple syrup (optional)

1 Tbsp fresh lemon juice

Pinch of black pepper

INSTRUCTIONS:

- In a small saucepan, bring water to a boil.
- Add turmeric, ginger, and black pepper, and reduce heat to a simmer for 10 minutes.
- Remove from heat and strain into cups.
- Stir in honey or maple syrup and lemon juice.
- Serve warm.

NUTRITIONAL FACTS (per Serving): Calories: 40 | Total Fat: 0g | Saturated Fat: 0g | Fiber: 1g | Protein: 0.5g | Carbohydrate: 10g of which sugars: 7g | Vitamin A: 0% DV | Vitamin C: 10% DV | Calcium: 2% DV | Iron: 2% DV

DETOXIFYING GREEN JUICE

A revitalizing and detoxifying green juice loaded with nutrients to cleanse your body and boost your energy levels.

INGREDIENTS:	PREP TIME: 10 min	COOK TIME: 0 min	SERVINGS: 2 Servings

INGREDIENTS:	
1 cucumber, peeled and chopped	**INSTRUCTIONS:** • Add all ingredients to a blender. • Blend until smooth. • Strain through a fine mesh sieve or nut milk bag if desired. • Serve immediately.
2 celery stalks, chopped	
1 green apple, chopped	
1 cup spinach leaves	
1/2 lemon, juiced	
1-inch piece of ginger, peeled	
1/2 cup parsley	
1 cup water	**NUTRITIONAL FACTS (per Serving):** Calories: 80 | Total Fat: 0.5g | Saturated Fat: 0g | Fiber: 4g | Protein: 2g | Carbohydrate: 18g of which sugars: 10g | Vitamin A: 50% DV | Vitamin C: 60% DV | Calcium: 6% DV | Iron: 6% DV

ANTI-CANDIDA STIR-FRY

A flavorful stir-fry packed with antifungal ingredients to help combat Candida and support overall health.

INGREDIENTS:	PREP TIME: 10 min	COOK TIME: 0 min	SERVINGS: 2 Servings

INGREDIENTS:	
1 Tbsp coconut oil	**INSTRUCTIONS:** • In a large skillet or wok, heat coconut oil over medium heat. Sauté onion and garlic until fragrant, about 3 minutes. • Add bell pepper, broccoli, mushrooms, zucchini, and snap peas. Stir-fry for 7-10 minutes until vegetables are tender-crisp. • Stir in coconut aminos, ground ginger, turmeric, salt, and pepper. • Cook for an additional 2-3 minutes, allowing flavors to meld. • Garnish with fresh cilantro and serve immediately.
1 onion, sliced	
2 cloves garlic, minced	
1 bell pepper, sliced	
1 cup broccoli florets	
1 cup sliced mushrooms	
1 zucchini, sliced	
1/2 cup snap peas	
2 Tbsp coconut aminos	
1 tsp ground ginger	
1/2 tsp turmeric	
Salt and pepper to taste	**NUTRITIONAL FACTS (per Serving):** Calories: 180 | Total Fat: 9g | Saturated Fat: 6g | Fiber: 6g | Protein: 4g | Carbohydrate: 22g of which sugars: 8g | Vitamin A: 60% DV | Vitamin C: 150% DV | Calcium: 6% DV | Iron: 10% DV
1/4 cup fresh cilantro, chopped	

Section III: The Meal Plan

Nourishing Your Body: A 4-Week Meal Plan Journey

This 4-week meal plan is your gateway to embracing Barbara O'Neill's holistic health principles through delicious, plant-based nutrition. Each day is thoughtfully designed with five meals: breakfast, mid-morning snack, lunch, afternoon snack, and dinner. This structure ensures a steady intake of nutrients and energy throughout your day.

By incorporating a variety of nutrient-dense, whole foods, this meal plan helps you explore new flavors and textures while promoting optimal health. You'll find recipes that span across different food groups, providing balanced nutrition without repeating the same main ingredients within a single day. This variety keeps your meals interesting and ensures you receive a wide range of vitamins, minerals, and antioxidants.

Following this plan offers numerous benefits. Expect improved digestion from fiber-rich meals, increased energy levels from balanced nutrients, and a stronger immune system from antioxidant-packed foods. Each recipe is crafted to support your body's natural healing processes, promoting overall well-being.

Dive into this meal plan and embark on a journey toward better health. Enjoy nourishing, flavorful meals that not only satisfy your taste buds but also contribute to your holistic wellness. Each day brings a new culinary adventure, helping you feel your best and thrive naturally.

		WEEK 1	WEEK 2
Day 1	Breakfast	Blueberry Oat Pancakes	Coconut Yogurt Parfait with Granola
	Snack	Apple Slices with Almond Butter	Spiced Pumpkin Seeds
	Lunch	Broccoli and Raisin Salad	Avocado and Corn Salad
	Snack	Roasted Garlic and Herb Cashews	Fresh Mango and Lime Salad
	Dinner	Baked Eggplant Parmesan	Vegan Lasagna with Cashew Cheese
Day 2	Breakfast	Flaxseed and Almond Granola	Apple Cinnamon Overnight Oats
	Snack	Coconut and Date Bliss Balls	Almond and Cranberry Trail Mix
	Lunch	Zucchini Noodles with Pesto and Cherry Tomatoes	Cauliflower Rice Stir-Fry with Tofu
	Snack	Fresh Pineapple and Mint Salad	Nut-Free Energy Bars
	Dinner	Lentil and Sweet Potato Shepherd's Pie	Black Bean and Butternut Squash Chili
Day 3	Breakfast	Avocado and Spinach Smoothie	Fresh Fruit Salad with Mint
	Snack	Edamame with Sea Salt	Baked Apple Chips with Cinnamon
	Lunch	Sweet Potato and Black Bean Tacos	Chickpea and Kale Stew
	Snack	Spiced Chickpea Snack	Healing Turmeric and Ginger Tea
	Dinner	Quinoa-Stuffed Bell Peppers	Protein-Packed Vegan Chili
Day 4	Breakfast	Lemon And Coconut Energy Balls	Turmeric and Ginger Smoothie
	Snack	Greek Yogurt with Honey and Walnuts	Edamame with Sea Salt
	Lunch	Lentil and Vegetable Soup	Beet And Arugula Salad with Goat Cheese
	Snack	Turmeric-Spiced Popcorn	Celery Sticks with Sunflower Seed Butter
	Dinner	Vegan Pad Thai with Tofu	Anti-Inflammatory Turmeric Soup
Day 5	Breakfast	Quinoa and Berry Breakfast Porridge	Warm Buckwheat Porridge with Berries
	Snack	Mixed Berry and Nut Energy Bars	Hummus with Carrot and Cucumber Sticks
	Lunch	Roasted Vegetable and Hummus Wrap	Grilled Portobello Mushroom Sandwich
	Snack	Celery Sticks with Sunflower Seed Butter	Roasted Garlic and Herb Cashews
	Dinner	Spinach and Chickpea Curry	Paleo Cauliflower Rice Bowl
Day 6	Breakfast	Almond Butter Banana Toast	Vegan Banana Nut Muffins
	Snack	Hummus with Carrot and Cucumber Sticks	Fresh Pineapple and Mint Salad
	Lunch	Baked Falafel with Tzatziki Sauce	Spaghetti Squash with Marinara Sauce
	Snack	Detoxifying Green Juice	Spiced Chickpea Snack
	Dinner	Stuffed Acorn Squash with Wild Rice	Vegan Pad Thai with Tofu
Day 7	Breakfast	Raw Cashew Cheesecake	Kale and Sweet Potato Hash
	Snack	Baked Zucchini Chips	Greek Yogurt with Honey and Walnuts
	Lunch	Mediterranean Stuffed Bell Peppers	Black Bean and Corn Salad with Lime Dressing
	Snack	Vegan Cheese and Cucumber Slices	Liver Detox Smoothie
	Dinner	Mushroom and Spinach Risotto	Vegan Lentil Loaf

		WEEK 3	WEEK 4
Day 1	Breakfast	Steel-Cut Oats with Mixed Nuts and Honey	Green Power Smoothie Bowl
	Snack	Coconut and Date Bliss Balls	Iced Hibiscus Tea
	Lunch	Hearty Vegetable and Barley Stew	Vegan Sushi Rolls with Avocado and Cucumber
	Snack	Baked Zucchini Chips	Vegan Cheese and Cucumber Slices
	Dinner	Mediterranean Quinoa Bowls	Quinoa-Stuffed Bell Peppers
Day 2	Breakfast	Carrot Cake Breakfast Bars	Chia Seed Pudding with Fresh Berries
	Snack	Fresh Mango and Lime Salad	Spiced Pumpkin Seeds
	Lunch	Eggplant and Lentil Moussaka	Black Bean and Corn Salad with Lime Dressing
	Snack	Spiced Pumpkin Seeds	Fresh Mango and Lime Salad
	Dinner	Creamy Coconut Lentil Curry	Stuffed Acorn Squash with Wild Rice
Day 3	Breakfast	Lemon and Chia Seed Scones	Sweet Potato and Black Bean Breakfast Burrito
	Snack	Spinach And Banana Smoothie	Baked Zucchini Chips
	Lunch	Wild Rice and Mushroom Pilaf	Roasted Beet and Quinoa Salad
	Snack	Anti-Inflammatory Golden Milk	Hummus with Carrot and Cucumber Sticks
	Dinner	Zucchini and Tomato Gratin	Vegan Lasagna with Cashew Cheese
Day 4	Breakfast	Spinach and Mushroom Breakfast Wrap	Coconut Yogurt Parfait with Granola
	Snack	Baked Apple Chips with Cinnamon	Edamame with Sea Salt
	Lunch	Carrot and Ginger Soup	Cucumber and Tomato Salad With Dill
	Snack	Turmeric-Spiced Popcorn	Spiced Chickpea Snack
	Dinner	Stuffed Portobello Mushrooms	Mediterranean Vegetable Tagine
Day 5	Breakfast	Dark Chocolate and Nut Clusters	Apple Cinnamon Overnight Oats
	Snack	Coconut Water and Berry Smoothie	Turmeric-Spiced Popcorn
	Lunch	Roasted Vegetable and Hummus Wrap	Zucchini Noodles with Pesto and Cherry Tomatoes
	Snack	Herbal Detox Tea	Celery Sticks with Sunflower Seed Butter
	Dinner	Dairy-Free Alfredo Pasta	Anti-Inflammatory Turmeric Soup
Day 6	Breakfast	Raw Chocolate Avocado Mousse	Blueberry And Chia Seed Pudding
	Snack	Mixed Berry and Nut Energy Bars	Fresh Pineapple and Mint Salad
	Lunch	Baked Falafel with Tzatziki Sauce	Spinach And Strawberry Salad
	Snack	Cucumber And Aloe Vera Juice	Almond and Cranberry Trail Mix
	Dinner	Lentil and Sweet Potato Shepherd's Pie	Black Bean and Butternut Squash Chili
Day 7	Breakfast	Vegan Scrambled Tofu with Vegetables	Raw Vegan Carrot Cake
	Snack	Apple Slices with Almond Butter	Mixed Berry and Nut Energy Bars
	Lunch	Chickpea and Kale Stew	Hearty Vegetable and Barley Stew
	Snack	Pineapple and Turmeric Smoothie	Roasted Garlic and Herb Cashews
	Dinner	Mushroom and Spinach Risotto	Creamy Coconut Lentil Curry

Conclusion

As you reach the conclusion of "The Dr. Barbara's Natural Healing Cookbook," you've embarked on a transformative journey toward optimal health and well-being. This book has provided you with a comprehensive guide to holistic nutrition, emphasizing the power of whole, plant-based foods, proper hydration, and mindful eating practices.

By embracing the recipes and principles shared within these pages, you are equipping yourself with the tools to nourish your body, boost your immune system, and support your natural healing processes. Whether you're starting your day with a nutrient-packed smoothie, enjoying a wholesome lunch, or indulging in a delicious yet healthy dessert, each meal is a step towards a healthier you.

The journey doesn't end here. Continue exploring and experimenting with the recipes, adapting them to your taste and lifestyle. Share your discoveries with others, inspiring them to embrace the benefits of natural, holistic eating. Remember, true health is a lifelong journey, and every choice you make brings you closer to a vibrant, energized, and balanced life.

Thank you for allowing this cookbook to be a part of your health journey. May it continue to inspire and guide you toward a path of natural healing and well-being. Enjoy the vibrant flavors and the nourishing benefits of each recipe, and embrace the positive changes they bring to your life. Here's to your health, happiness, and vitality!

Printed in the USA
CPSIA information can be obtained
at www.ICGtesting.com
CBHW081844171124
17565CB00013B/214